yogapilates

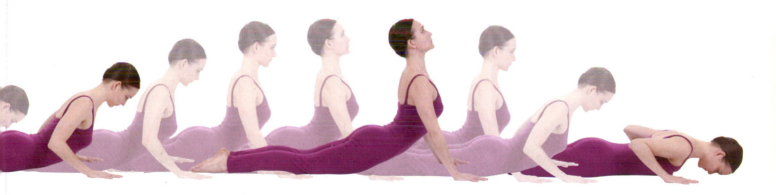

a *flow*motion™ title

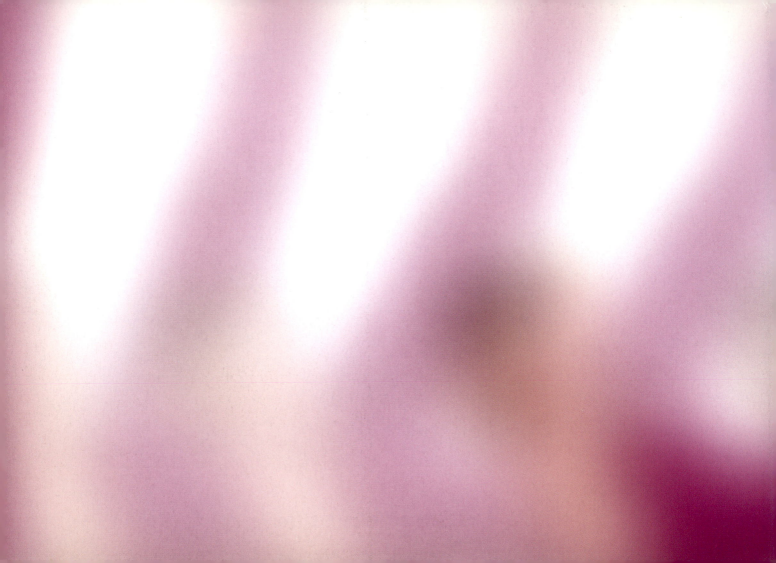

yogapilates

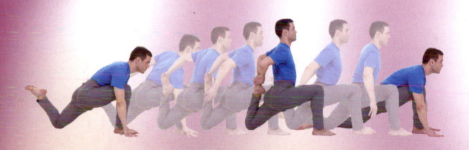

diana holland

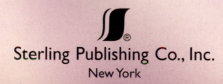

Sterling Publishing Co., Inc.

New York

Created and conceived by
Axis Publishing Limited
8c Accommodation Road
London NW11 8ED
www.axispublishing.co.uk

Creative Director: Siân Keogh
Editorial Director: Brian Burns
Project Designer: Axis Design Editions
Project Editor: Conor Kilgallon
Production Manager: Tim Clarke
Photographer: Mike Good

Library of Congress Cataloging-in-Publication Data
Available

10 9 8 7 6 5 4 3 2 1

Published in 2003 by Sterling Publishing Co., Inc.
387 Park Avenue South, New York, NY 10016
Text and images © Axis Publishing Limited 2003
Distributed in Canada by Sterling Publishing
C/o Canadian Manda Group,
One Atlantic Avenue, Suite 105
Toronto, Ontario, Canada, M6K 3E7

ISBN 1–4027–0904–8

Printed by Star Standard (Pte) Limited

Models: Leonidas Mezilis and Ngio Ballard. Trousers worn
by Leonidas were kindly supplied by Niketown, London.
All other clothes were kindly supplied by Sansha, London.
Many thanks to Michelle McKenna.

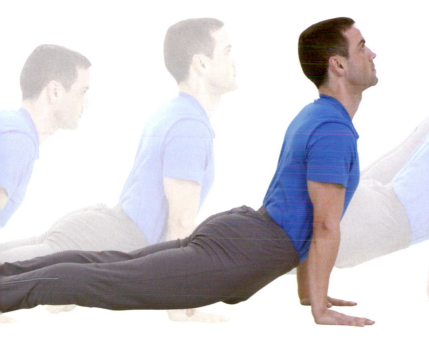

a *flowmotion*™ title

yogapilates

contents

introduction

yoga

Yoga as a philisophy and form of exercise has been around for over 5,000 years and was first practiced by seers and Rishis (forest dwellers) in northern India. Described as "the stilling of the through waves of the mind," the traditions of this ancient practice have found an important niche in today's busy world. Yoga now, as then, is a powerful form of support, helping people cope with the stresses of modern life.

The many yoga postures also create a strong and supple body, which improves overall physical health. Yoga exercises help flush toxins from the body, improve blood circulation, and keep all the internal bodily processes functioning smoothly. Yoga breathing has the power to calm the mind, releasing tension and offering inner peace. Compared with many other exercise systems, yoga moves at at slower, more mindful pace, focusing on flowing breathing and movement to connect mind and body.

pilates

Joseph Pilates developped his exercise system in the early 1900s. Although he was relatively unknown during his lifetime, his system is one of the most popular forms of training. The pilates method is a complete system of exercises designed to give you strength, flexibility, coordination, correct body alignment, and a unity of mind, body, and spirit. At the heart of this technique is the development of powerful abdominals—the center body.

YOGA BREATHING AND PERFECT POSE

Some of the exercises shown in this book require yoga breathing, others, pilates breathing (see opposite). To practice yoga breathing, sit tall on a firm cushion, keeping your chest and shoulders relaxed and your abdominals pulled in. Bring your right foot to your groin so the top of your foot is on the floor. Do the same with your left foot and place it in front of your right. Rest your hands on your knees. This is perfect pose. Inhale fully through your nose, feeling your ribs expand sideways. Then exhale slowly through your nose, feeling your ribs softly contract. As you inhale and exhale, allow your breath to gently resonate at the back of your throat, creating a soft sound like that of a distant sea. This is called Victorious Breath.

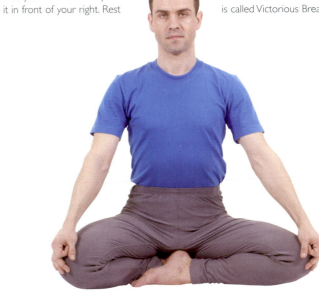

yoga pilates fusion

The fusion of both systems produces flowing, rhythmic, choreographed exercise routines that entwine in a unique, challenging system. This system works to create all-over body strength, stamina, flexibility, good alignment, deeper breathing, and firm abdominals.

The routines target all areas of mind and body fitness. You will gain physical strength from practicing yoga pilates fusion exercises, but your development will be in keeping with your own body proportions. You will not overdevelop arm or leg muscles, but rather strengthen and lengthen your whole body the way it is. This doesn't mean that you won't change your shape—you certainly will if you do the work out daily and look at and change your lifestyle and eating habits to more healthy ones. Even if you only work out two or three times a week, you should soon begin to notice an improvement in your posture and your physical stamina.

The human body was designed to move, but many people today live very sedentary lives, sitting in cars, in front of computers, and slouching in front of the television. This lifestyle leads to weak and untoned muscles. Also, muscular movement contributes a great deal to the circulatory system of the body. The contraction of our muscles helps pump blood back to the heart as well as moving the lymphs (tissue-bathing fluids) around our bodies. A sedentary lifestyle can produce weak circulation.

Yoga pilates fusion exercises bring balance back into the body and teach us to stand tall, lifting up against gravity. But you need muscle

PILATES BREATHING

Sit tall with your legs crossed ("easy pose"), resting your hands on the sides of your ribs. Keeping your shoulders relaxed and your abdominals pulled in, inhale fully through your nose, feeling your back and side ribs expand sideways, gently pushing against your hands. Slowly and fully exhale through the mouth as if you were gently blowing out a candle. Feel your side ribs gently sink back down. Practice this breathing for a minute or two before starting your yoga pilates fusion exercises.

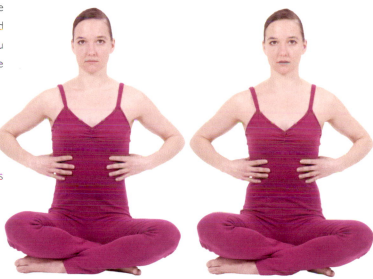

tone to do this. Untoned muscles do not adequately support your skeleton, and this can lead to pain and stiffness in your joints. Good muscle tone helps us stand, sit, move, and breathe with ease and grace, and when the spine is strong and flexible the diaphragm works more efficiently, making us more capable of fuller, deeper breathing.

Yoga pilates fusion exercises build slowly throughout the book, so you will not be putting undue wear and tear on your body. The kind of exercises involved build muscular stamina while strengthening the heart and lungs slowly and carefully. While following the sequences, you will be working in very specific ways by concentrating on particular movements combined with coordinated breathing and mental focus. Attention to accuracy is needed, but you will achieve an enormous sense of satisfaction as you progress and see your body become fitter and more toned and your overall health improve.

If you stay with the yoga pilates fusion training, its effects will spill over into your daily life. Your posture will change, giving you more confidence

NEUTRAL SPINE

It is important to achieve the correct posture for a neutral spine. The first two pictures show incorrect positions; the third shows the correct pose.

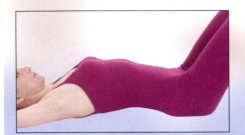

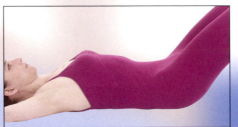

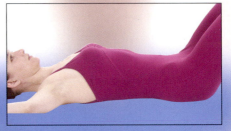

The position shown here is incorrect because the spine is over-arching, the pelvis is tilting forward, and the abdominals are not engaged.

Things have also gone wrong here because the spine is flat and the pelvis is tilted up at the front, with the result that there is no lumbar curve.

This is the correct alignment, maintaining the natural curves of your spine. Also, the pelvic floor muscles are lifting and the abdominal muscles are drawing in, engaging the muscles around the spine and lower abdomen. All your movements should radiate out from this stable center.

and courage to face the world and your breathing will deepen, generating vital energy in the body and unlocking tension. Altogether, you will be more relaxed, focused, and positive.

center body

In yoga pilates fusion, creating a strong, stable, center body is very important, since it is from here that you control all your movements. Your physical center comprises the muscles that wrap around your lower torso —the deeper abdominal muscles and the muscles of the pelvic floor.

To get a sense of your center, practice the following exercise daily. Lie on your back with your knees bent, your feet and legs hip width apart, your neck and shoulders relaxed, and your face soft. Place your hands on your lower abdomen. Focus on the natural rhythm of your breathing, following your breath in and out of your body. Then gently breathe in, and as you breathe out, draw the lower part of your abdomen in toward your spine. Hold this contraction as you smoothly and steadily breathe in and out.

pelvic floor

The pelvic floor is the term used to describe the layers of muscles that lie within the pelvis, forming its base. These muscles extend inside your body from your lower sacrum and coccyx at the back, to the pubic bone at the front, like a hammock. The pelvic floor muscles need to support the contents of your abdomen and resist the pull of gravity. A weak pelvic floor can cause vital energy to be lost, causing tiredness and even depression.

BEFORE YOU START

If you are certain you are medically healthy, you can begin your yoga pilates fusion straight away, but if you have any doubts, seek medical advice first. Also seek medical advice if you suffer from severe stiffness or any back, knee, or neck problems. Do not start any exercise program if you have any serious medical condition. Also:

■ Find a place that is warm, clean, and private. Wear comfortable clothes that breathe and that you can easily move in. Work on a nonslip mat. If you choose to play music, pick something that stays in the background with a soft flowing tempo.

■ Practice the exercises in the order in which they are presented. Yoga pilates fusion is choreographed and should be done as a flowing sequence. If you are a beginner, stick to the beginner's exercises and only move on as your stamina and technique improve. Don't try to race ahead.

■ It is not advisable to start an exercise program if you are pregnant.

■ Do not eat at least two to three hours before you exercise.

■ Start slowly so your body gets used to moving correctly. Never force your body to do something it is not able to do—stop if you feel pain. Leave that exercise out and get advice from an experienced teacher.

■ Don't hold your breath; keep your breathing smooth and even. The general rule is to exhale as you go into a movement and to inhale as you come out of that movement.

■ Don't miss out the relaxation sequence at the end of the class. Make sure that you are warm and comfortable. Place a folded towel under your head and a blanket over your body.

exercises and stretches

pelvic floor exercises

CONTRACT AND RELEASE

Try to practice these exercises, which can be done lying or sitting down at least three times a day. To start with, focus on the pelvic floor. Tighten and draw the muscles up as you breathe in then release them slowly as you breathe out. Repeat four times. Then draw the muscles up as you breathe in. Hold them tight while you inhale and exhale again. Then let them go slowly as you breathe out.

QUICK TEMPO EXERCISE

Lift and tighten and let go in quick succession while breathing normally and repeat 10 to 15 times. Once you have control over your deep abdominal muscles and muscles of your pelvic floor, keep them engaged throughout the sequences and use them to initiate every movement.

RECLINING COBBLER

This soothing stretch increases flexibility in your hips and groin and gently opens the chest.

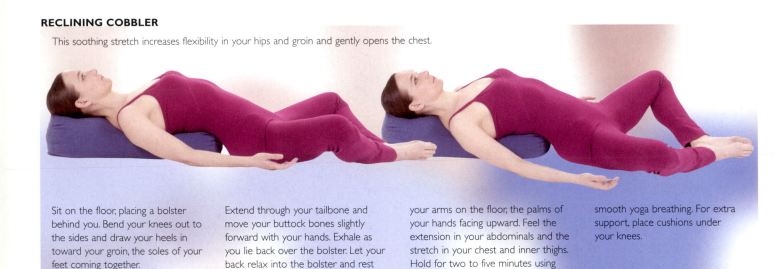

Sit on the floor, placing a bolster behind you. Bend your knees out to the sides and draw your heels in toward your groin, the soles of your feet coming together.

Extend through your tailbone and move your buttock bones slightly forward with your hands. Exhale as you lie back over the bolster. Let your back relax into the bolster and rest

your arms on the floor, the palms of your hands facing upward. Feel the extension in your abdominals and the stretch in your chest and inner thighs. Hold for two to five minutes using

smooth yoga breathing. For extra support, place cushions under your knees.

body posture—mountain pose

Your body posture reveals your feelings to the outside world and also produces feelings within you. If you stand badly, knees dropped in, tummy out, back and shoulders rounded, you will not only start to feel terrible, but your discomfort and awkwardness will be eveident in your movements. With a little training you could stand properly, feeling and looking a lot better.

The way to improve poor body posture is to start by thinking tall and standing straight. Lift the soles of your feet and stretch them up from the center of your arches and then press them down into the floor, stretching your toes. Now raise your heels from the center of your arches and put them down again. Keep the weight even on the inner and outer edges of both feet, the heels and the soles of the feet and then lift your insteps. From this firm base, lift your inner and outer ankle bones. Stretch your legs up as long as you can. Draw your tailbone down and in so your pelvis is sitting straight on the tops of your thighs. Lift up out of your hips. Lift and stretch your spine, lifting your abdomen and keeping both sides of your waist long. Lift your side and back ribs. Open your chest and make your upper back wide. Relax your shoulders and draw them down. Then relax your arms and hands, letting them hang naturally down the side of your body. Stretch your neck up, long and easy, keeping the throat soft. Keep your head straight and your chin at right angles to your breastbone.

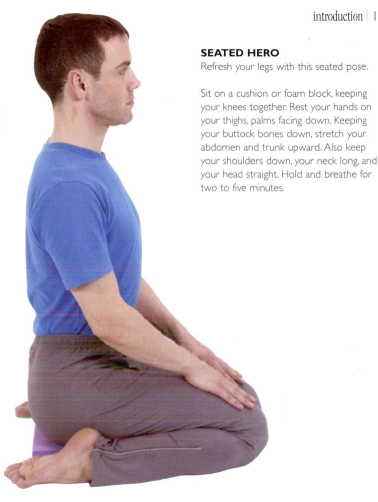

SEATED HERO
Refresh your legs with this seated pose.

Sit on a cushion or foam block, keeping your knees together. Rest your hands on your thighs, palms facing down. Keeping your buttock bones down, stretch your abdomen and trunk upward. Also keep your shoulders down, your neck long, and your head straight. Hold and breathe for two to five minutes.

Soften and relax the face and look ahead with a soft gaze. Breathe easy. Practice this pose, the mountain pose, with your feet and legs together (if this is difficult, stand with your feet and legs slightly apart). This may seem like a lot to remember just to stand up, but persevere because all your standing work will start from this important position.

the sequences

The opening sequences in the book are simple floor exercises to bring self-awareness and attention to your body and start a connection with your center body. These are followed by standing fusion sequences that will boost your energy and strengthen and open the whole body while stimulating internal organs and vital body systems. The standing sequences should be done dynamically with full extension of the limbs and the trunk. Keep your breathing flowing as you move smoothly from one position to the next. The same principles should be applied to the balancing poses, which will help you achieve control over your body and strengthen your coordination and concentration. The backbends are rejuvenating—they give you energy and courage by opening the chest and bringing flexibility to the spine. The twists are very effective at bringing relief to backaches, neck, and headaches and they massage the internal organs, improving kidney and liver functions. They also improve digestion and help reduce fat around the waist.

The final section is floor work exercises, which are done sitting, lying, and kneeling. Working on the floor has the advantage of allowing you to isolate and directly work on specific muscle groups.

RECLINING HERO

This pose stretches the front of the hips, the thighs, and the abdomen. It is also a very restful pose.

Sit between your feet, your buttocks on the floor. Exhale and lean back, placing your elbows on the floor first. Move your elbows out and stretch your trunk over the bolster, extending through the tailbone. Keep your arms relaxed, palms facing upward. Keep your chest open and your face relaxed. Hold and breathe for three to five minutes. Inhale as you come up out of the pose.

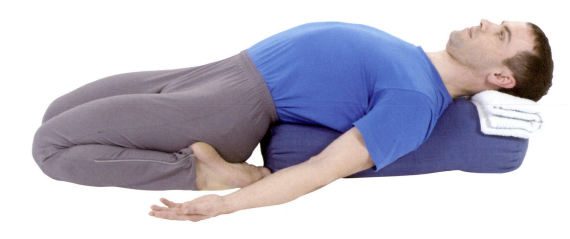

breathing

Breathing is the key to linking your mind and body—concentrating on a smooth, flowing breath will bring fluid, rhythmic movement. Thus rhythmic breathing threads your movements together. When you exhale fully, you expel stale air and gases from the bottom of your lungs; when you inhale fully, you replenish your body with fresh air that energizes and revitalizes your system.

Practice your breathing lying or sitting down with your eyes closed. First, exhale fully, expelling all air from your lungs. Then gently inhale through your nostrils, gradually lengthening the breath without straining. If you strain, you will get tense—it is important that you stay relaxed. Encourage the breath to move laterally (sideways) into the back and side ribs and diaphragm. Feel your ribcage gradually expand, the lower ribs opening first. Keep your neck and shoulders relaxed. Pause naturally for a second. Then breathe out slowly and completely, also through the nose. Take a natural pause; then breathe in again through your nose. Each breath should be smooth and steady with even lengths. Do theese five to ten minutes and practice daily—even on the bus.

KNEE HUGGING

Knee hugging gently stretches the back and loosens the hips. Use yoga breathing.

Lie on your back, your legs extended and your arms resting on the floor by your sides. Lift your right leg. Interlock your hands and place them on the top of your right shin and gently hug your knee to your chest. Hold for five breaths and then change to the left leg. Repeat the sequence again.

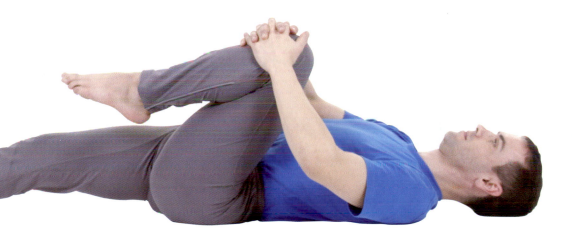

TIPS FOR BEGINNERS

You may find it useful to use equipment or adjust your body to achieve some of the positions.

- If you find it difficult to bend forward because your hamstrings are tight or your lower back is stiff, bend your knees to start with while doing the standing forward bends.

- If your hamstrings are tight in the sitting forward bends and you find it impossible to catch your feet, loop a belt around your feet and just extend and lift your spine—don't move into the forward bend.

- If your back is stiff in the seated positions, sit on a cushion or folded blankets. This will help you get a better lift through your hips and spine, helping you achieve the seated twist and forward bends.

- If you have trouble extending and lifting your legs off the floor in the back strengthener exercise, place a thick rolled-up towel under your thighs.

- If it is uncomfortable to sit on the floor with your knees bent out to the side, place cushions underneath them for support.

- In standing balances like the eagle and half moon, you can help yourself to balance by supporting your back against a wall. Similarly with the dancer balance, place your hand against a wall instead of extending your arms up toward the ceiling.

- If you do not feel the stretch in your spine in the downward facing dog position because your weight is too far forward on your arms (usually due to tight shoulders, hips, or hamstrings), bend your knees slightly while in the pose, but remember to keep lifting your hips high to the ceiling.

- To ease the stretch in side standing postures, such as triangle pose, place a block or brick beside you. This will help you reach the floor. Remember, though, to keep extending up through your supporting arm.

- If you feel discomfort lying on your back, place a small cushion or folded towel underneath your head and a thick rolled-up towel or bolster underneath your knees.

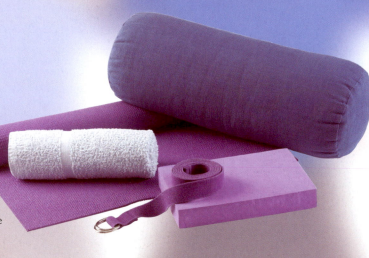

NECK RELEASE

The neck release warms and loosens your neck muscles before you start your exercises. It is important to move your neck smoothly.

Sit with the soles of your feet together, about 2½ft (0.75m) away from your body. Keep your abdominals drawn in. Lower your arms to your sides, your fingers on the floor. Sit tall with your shoulders down, gazing ahead. Inhale.

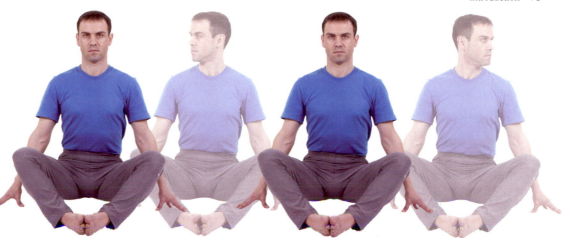

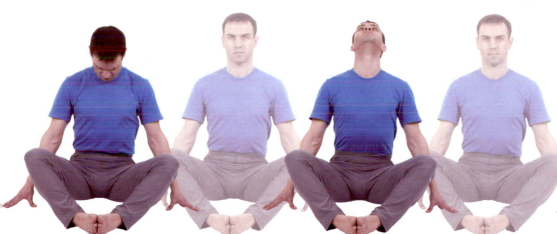

Exhale as you look to your right; inhale as you look ahead; exhale as you look to your left; inhale as you look ahead; exhale as you look down; inhale as you look ahead; exhale as you lift your face to the ceiling, being careful not to let your head drop back; inhale and look ahead to finish.

SEATED SIDE BENDS

This exercise integrates movement and breathing. Bending sideways also stretches the muscles between the ribs, encouraging deeper breathing. This is a yoga breathing exercise.

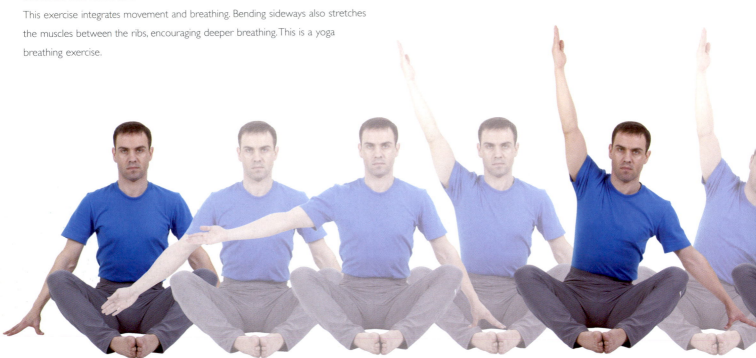

Sit tall with the soles of your feet together, your abdominals drawn in, and your arms extending down to your sides.

Using your breath to motivate the movement, inhale and float your right arm above your head, with the palms turning upward.

Keep your shoulders down and your neck long and easy. Keep your hips anchored into the floor and your trunk facing forward.

Exhale as you curve your torso slowly over to the left, extending your right arm over as well. Keep your shoulder blades flat against your back.

Inhale, using your breath to lift your arm and torso back to an upright position.

Exhale as you lower your right arm and come back to sitting tall. Keep your shoulders relaxed and your face soft.

Remember that your arms are extensions of your back. Try to feel this connection as you lift and extend your arms.

Repeat the exercise on the other side. Carry out the sequence twice on each side.

DANCE CONTRACTION

The dance contraction is a deep flowing movement that energizes the body. The strong pull back tones the abdominals and stretches the spine. This is a pilates breathing exercise.

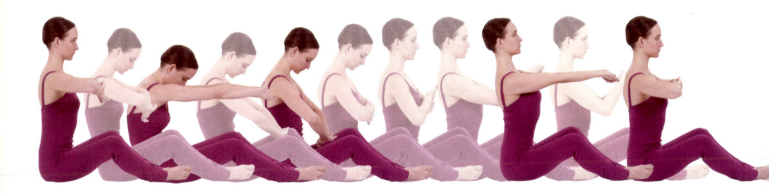

Sit tall with the soles of your feet together, your knees out to the sides. Interlock your fingers with your palms facing inward. Lift your elbows to shoulder height and inhale.

As you exhale, start the contraction by tilting your pelvis under and scooping your abdominals back, curving your spine outward. Push your hands forward, palms turning outward.

Inhale as you begin to straighten your spine, starting with your pelvis and working up your back. Move your hands in toward your body, turning your palms inward.

Keep exhaling as you complete the lift. Turn your hands so your palms lift up and turn outward. Repeat the contraction three more times. Inhale to finish in the starting position; then exhale and lower your arms.

go with the flow

The special Flowmotion images used in this book have been created to ensure that you can see each stage of every exercise and not just isolated highlights. Each sequence is shown across the page from left to right, demonstrating how the move progresses and develops safely and effectively, and is accompanied by clear, concise step-by-step captions.

Below this, another layer of information in the timeline breaks the move into its various key stages, with instructions indicating when to "inhale," "exhale," and "breathe normally." The symbols in the timeline also include instructions for when to pause and hold a position and when to move seamlessly from one stage to the next.

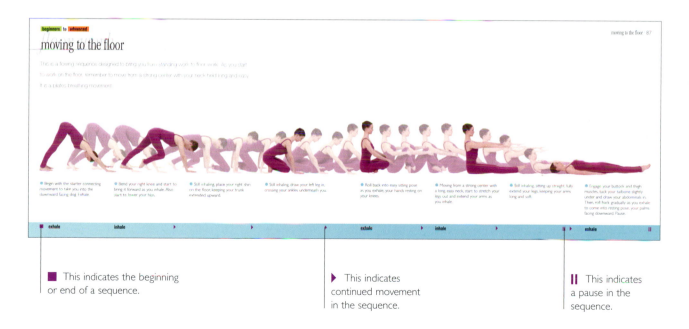

beginners to **advanced**

moving to the floor

moving to the floor 87

This is a flowing sequence designed to bring you from standing work to floor work. As you start to work on the floor, remember to move from a strong center with your neck held long and easy. It is a pilates breathing movement.

- Begin with the starter connecting movement to take you into the downward facing dog. Exhale.
- Bend your right knee and start to bring it forward as you inhale. Also start to lower your hips.
- Still inhaling, place your right shin on the floor, keeping your trunk extended upward.
- Still inhaling, draw your left leg in, crossing your ankles underneath you.
- Roll back into easy sitting pose in you exhale, your hands resting on your knees.
- Moving from a strong center with a long, easy neck, start to stretch your legs out and extend your arms as you inhale.
- Still inhaling, sitting up straight, fully extend your legs, keeping your arms long and soft.
- Engage your buttock and thigh muscles, tuck your tailbone slightly under and draw your abdominals in. Then, roll back gradually as you exhale to come into resting pose, your palms facing downward. Pause.

exhale inhale ▶ ▶ ▶ exhale ▶ inhale ▶ ❚❚ ▶ exhale ❚❚

■ This indicates the beginning or end of a sequence.

▶ This indicates continued movement in the sequence.

❚❚ This indicates a pause in the sequence.

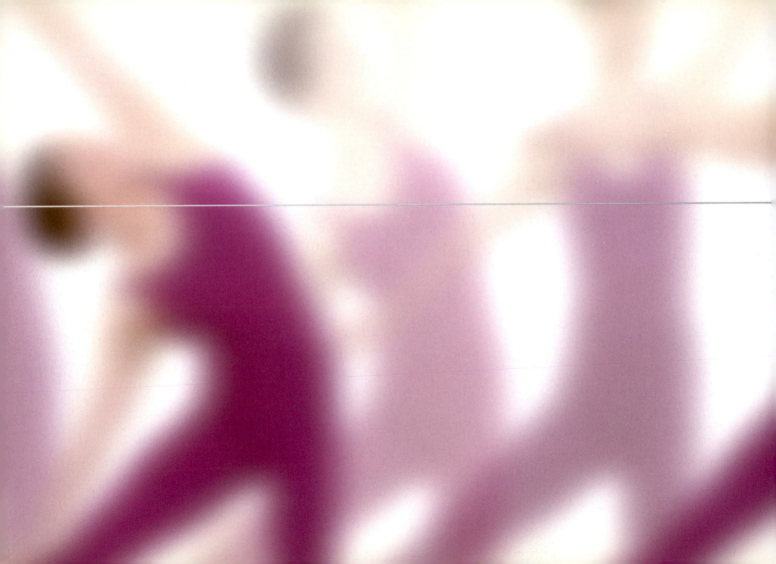

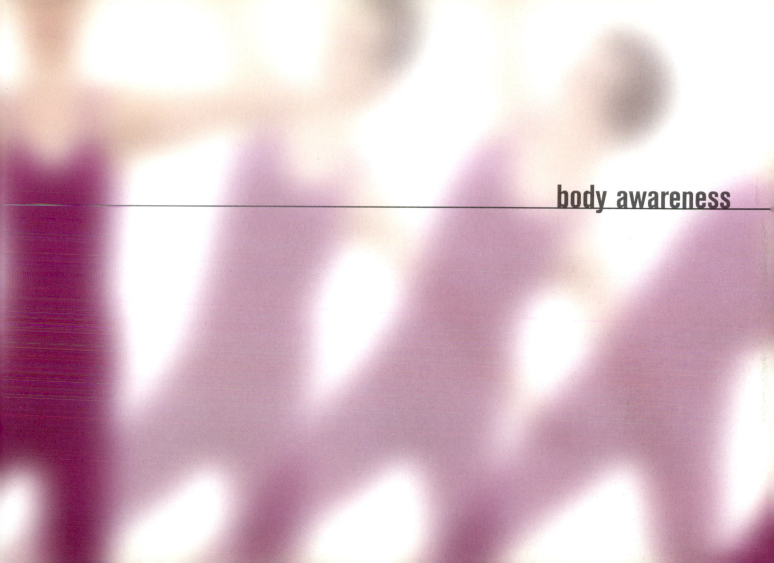

body awareness

moving bridge

This is a simple warm-up for the back that also firms the back of the legs, buttocks, and abdomen.

It also eases lower back pain. This is a pilates breathing exercise.

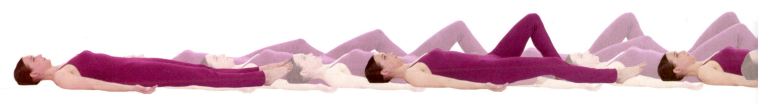

● Lie on your back, your arms by your sides, palms facing up (the "corpse," or resting, pose). Make sure you are completely relaxed and let go of all your cares. Focus on your breathing.

● Lift your pelvic floor, drawing your abdomen toward your spine. Keep a long, easy neck.

● As you inhale, draw your legs up, one at a time, your knees pointing at the ceiling. Turn the palms of your hands to face the floor.

● Make sure your feet and legs are parallel to each other, hip width apart. Feel your inner ankles, inner shins, and inner thighs drawing toward the pelvic floor.

inhale

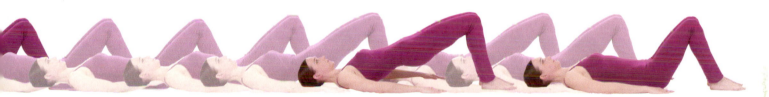

● Start to peel your lower and upper back, sacrum, and tailbone smoothly off the floor as you exhale. Your hips should now be completely off the floor. This is the bridge.

● Inhale as you hold the bridge. Make sure your feet are pressing firmly into the floor and engage your inner thigh muscles. Draw your pelvic floor up and keep your abdomen long and flat. Also keep a long, easy neck.

● Start to come down smoothly as you exhale, placing your upper and lower back, sacrum, and tailbone on the floor.

● Inhale as you hold the neutral position. Then repeat the lift four times, exhaling as you lift.

exhale ▶ **inhale** ▶ **exhale** ▶ **inhale and exhale** ‖

simple abdominals

This exercise works all the major abdominal muscles. It also flattens the tummy, tones the waist, and strengthens the pelvic floor. This is a pilates breathing exercise.

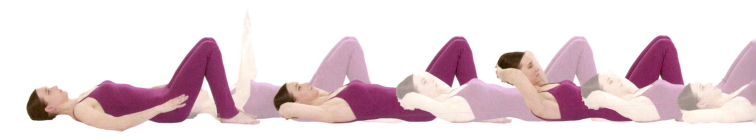

● Continue from the position on the previous page. Bring both hands back behind your head and interlock your fingers. Keep your neck long and soft and your elbows slightly off the floor so you can see them out of the corner of your eyes.

● With your hips in the neutral position and your shoulder blades drawing down the back, prepare to lift your body as you inhale. Feel your pelvic floor lifting and your abdomen drawing down.

● Start to lift as you exhale, lifting your head and shoulders off the floor. Keep your neck and shoulders relaxed, and avoid pulling on your neck.

● Hold as you inhale.

▶ **inhale** ▶ **exhale** ▶ **inhale** ‖ ▶

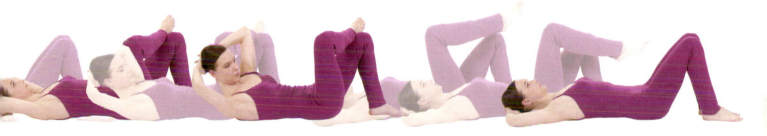

● Come back down as you exhale. Repeat the sequence four to eight times.

● Inhale as you lift your right foot onto your left knee. Keep your hips stable.

● As you exhale, lift your head and shoulders, turning from the waist. Lift your left elbow toward your right knee and be careful not to pull on your neck. Hold as you inhale.

● Come back down smoothly as you exhale. Repeat four to eight times on one side; then swap your legs over and repeat on the other side. When you have finished, lower your legs back to the starting point.

exhale ‖ ▶ inhale ▶ exhale and inhale ‖ ▶ exhale ‖

single leg raise

body awareness

This exercise encourages core stability and strengthens the abdomen and legs. It also brings awareness to your center. Focus on keeping your pelvis still as you work your leg. This is a pilates breathing exercise.

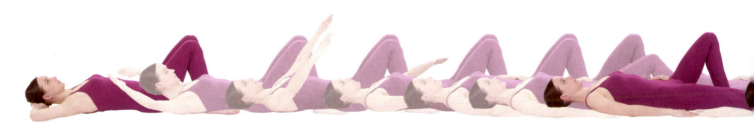

● Continue from the position on the previous page.

● Release your hands from behind your head as you inhale and bring your left hand down to your abdomen, fingers spreading. Place your right hand down alongside your body. Keep your legs parallel and your hips and lower back in a neutral position.

● Draw your abdominal muscles down as you exhale. Then inhale as you press your right foot down and along the floor and stretch out the leg, flexing the foot.

● Float the extended leg off the floor toward the ceiling as you exhale. Keep extending through the heel.

▶ **inhale** ▶ **exhale and inhale** ▶ **exhale** ▶

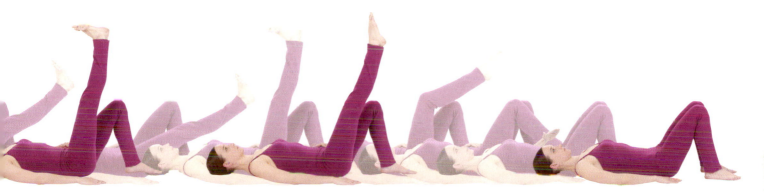

● Draw your abdominals down. Inhale as you lower your right leg to just above hip level, making sure your sacrum and lower back are still pressing into the floor, with your abdominals engaged. Exhale as you float your leg back up. Repeat three times.

● Inhale as you point your foot.

● Bend your leg and put your foot back on the floor as you exhale.

● Pause, breathe normally, and repeat on the other side.

inhale and exhale ❙❙ ▶ inhale ▶ exhale ▶ breathe normally ❙❙

roll-ups *awareness*

This movement works the abdominal muscles, massages the spine, and improves balance. Remember to fully engage your pelvic floor and abdominal muscles as you move. This is a pilates breathing exercise.

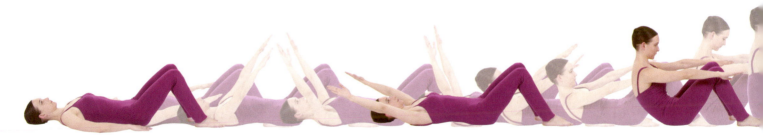

● Continue from the position on the previous page.

● Extend your arms over your head as you inhale.

● Drawing your shoulder blades down your back, engage your pelvic floor and abdomen as you exhale.

● As you inhale, start to float your arms forward, bringing your chin to your chest, and exhale as you peel your spine off the floor, little by little.

▶   **inhale**   ▶   **exhale**   ▶   **inhale and exhale**   ▶

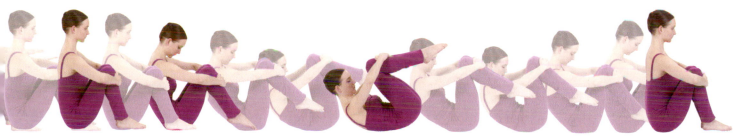

● Inhale as you come up to a sitting position, eyes gazing straight ahead, hands on shins.

● Draw your abdominals back and curl your body like a ball as you exhale.

● Roll backward with momentum as you inhale; then roll back to an upright position as you exhale. Repeat four to six times.

● Finish in a sitting position, with your hands resting on your shins and your shoulders relaxed with a long, easy neck.

inhale　▶　**exhale**　▶　**inhale and exhale**　❚❚ ▶　❚❚

easy pose *awareness*

This is a good, simple stretch for the upper spine and chest. As the movement progresses,

the stretch moves into the hips and buttocks. This is a yoga breathing exercise.

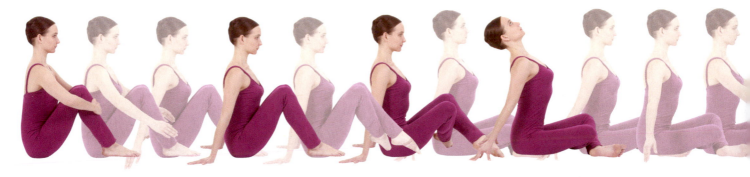

● Continue from the position on the previous page.

● Place your hands behind your back, keeping your torso lifted.

● Cross your legs with your right shin in front of your left shin, your right heel in front of your left knee, and your left foot under your right knee. Inhale as you do so.

● Lift your chest toward the ceiling, opening it up as you exhale. Be careful not to throw your head back.

▶ **breathe normally** ▶ **inhale** ▶ **exhale** ▶

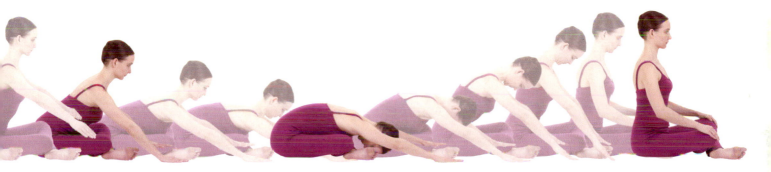

● Come out of this position as you inhale; then hinging from your hips, move forward and place your hands on the floor in front of you, spreading your fingers and palms into the ground.

● Keep your sitting bones and your buttocks anchored into the floor, your abdominals drawn in, and your chest open. Slide further down, folding forward as you exhale. Hold this forward bend for five breaths.

● Making sure your abdominals are still drawn in, start to bring your body back up to a sitting position, inhaling as you do so.

● Sitting upright, keep your spine lifted and your neck long and easy. Gaze straight ahead. Place your hands on your knees.

inhale ▶ **exhale** ▶ **inhale** ▶ **breathe normally** ❙❙

cat and dogtail

This simple warm-up exercise will improve your spinal flexibility and help flatten your tummy.

Move smoothly from one position to another. Use yoga breathing.

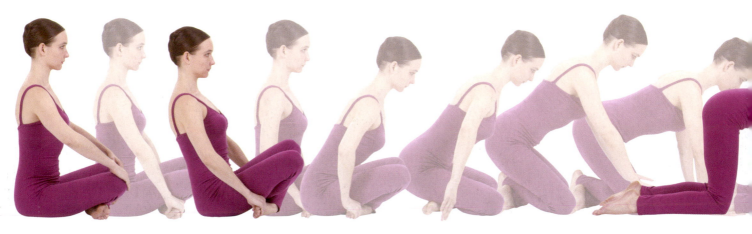

● Continue from the position on the previous page.

● Catch your feet with your hands and pull them back under your hips, tilting back slightly and inhaling as you do so.

● Drawing your abdominals in strongly, push down on your feet with your hands, and, with momentum, propel yourself forward onto your hands and knees as you exhale.

● Make sure your hands and knees are parallel to each other, hip width apart, and your hands are directly under your shoulders, fingers and palms spreading into the floor. Your back should be flat like a table top, your hips and thighs at right angles.

▶   **inhale**   ▶   **exhale**   ▶   **inhale**   ▶

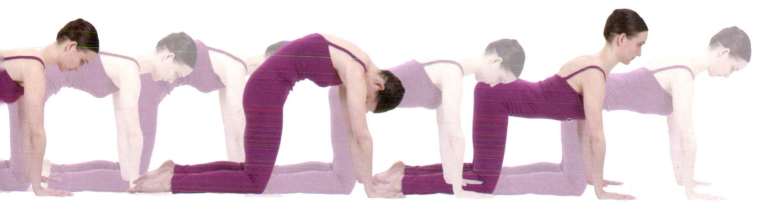

● Draw your abdominals in as you exhale. Tuck your tailbone under and start to drop your chin. Start to push your spine toward the ceiling.

● Still exhaling, push your spine toward the ceiling, arched like a cat's back. Keep your inner thighs drawing up, pelvic floor lifting, and feel the stretch across the upper back and shoulders, head heavy.

● Inhale as you move out of the cat pose, extending your tailbone away, lengthening your abdomen, and lifting your sternum and chin. Arch your spine the other way to form the dogtail as you inhale. Repeat both the cat and dogtail three more times.

● Move smoothly back into the table top position, breathing normally.

exhale ▶   ▶ **inhale**   ‖ ▶   **breathe normally**   ‖

wrist and toe stretches

Wrist stretches loosen stiff fingers, hands, and wrists and are good for people who use computer keyboards frequently. Toe stretches extend and stretch the soles of the feet and promote suppleness in the toes and strong arches. They also bring relief to aching feet. This is a yoga breathing exercise.

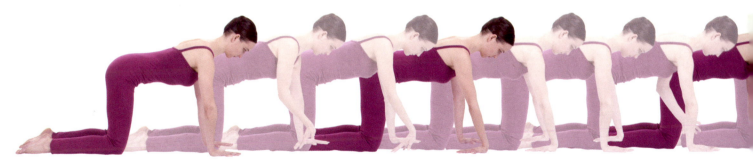

● Continue from the position on the previous page.

● Turn your hands outward, one at a time, fingers pointing toward your knees. Exhale as you do so. Hold for five breaths.

● Turn your hands back to the starting position, one at a time as you inhale. Remember to keep your abdomen long and lifted so your back stays straight.

● Starting with your right hand, turn and place the back of your hand on the floor, fingers pointing toward your left hand. Do not put any body weight on the bent wrist. Draw up through the wrists and elbows of both arms. Hold for three to five breaths.

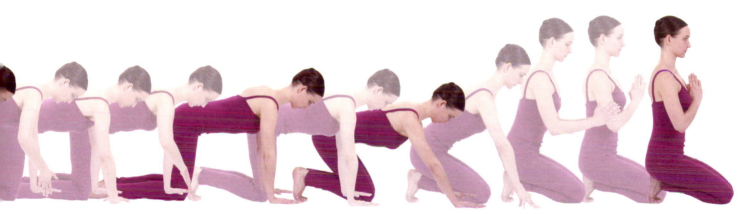

● Inhale as you put your right hand back on the floor, palm down. Repeat with the left hand. Finish in a neutral position, both palms spreading into the floor.

● Place your legs together, tuck your toes under, and draw your abdominals in. Drop your hips onto your heels as you exhale.

● Come up to a kneeling position as you inhale, hands together. Keep your spine lifted, your neck long and easy, and your eyes closed. Relax and focus on your breathing. Hold for five to ten smooth breaths.

● Lean forward slightly, release your toes, and sit back again with your hips on your heels. Also bring your palms together in front of your chest, resting your thumbs on your breast bone and keeping your elbows down and relaxed. This is the prayer pose.

inhale ▶ exhale ▶ inhale ❚❚ ▶ breathe normally ❚❚

gate*body awareness*

This lovely long side stretch firms and lengthens the waist,

stretches the rib cage, and encourages full, deep breathing.

It also stretches the spine. Use yoga breathing.

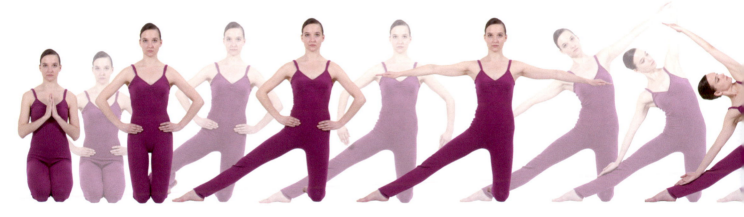

● Continue from the position on the previous page. Then, breathing normally, rise up and place your hands on your hips, drawing your leg muscles up and lifting your pelvic floor. Keep your abdomen long and lifted and open your chest.

● From a strong center, extend your right leg out to the side, keeping your left hip directly over your left knee. Align your right heel with your left knee. Breathe normally.

● Float your arms up to shoulder height as you inhale and extend through the elbows, wrists, and fingers. Rotate your hands smoothly so your palms face the ceiling.

● Lower the back of your right hand onto your right shin, extending your left arm over your head. Exhale as you do so. Slowly turn your head to look past the inside of your left arm at the ceiling. Hold for three to five breaths.

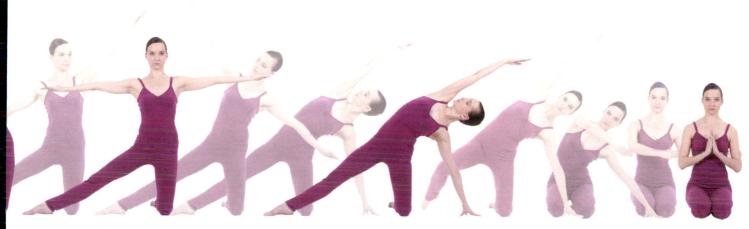

● From a firm base and strong center, come back up to an upright position as you inhale, turning your arms so your palms face downward.

● Moving from a strong center, exhale as you lower your left hand toward the floor and extend your right arm over your head. Hold for three to five breaths and finish on an inbreath.

● Curl your body forward as you exhale, keeping your pelvic floor lifted and abdomen drawing in. Sit on your heels.

● Inhale as you gently bring your hands into prayer pose, lifting your spine and relaxing your shoulders, keeping a soft gaze straight ahead. Breathe normally; then repeat on the other side.

inhale ▶ exhale and inhale ❚❚ ▶ exhale ▶ inhale ❚❚

downward dog with walkback

The downward dog builds strength in the back, legs, arms, and abdominal muscles. It is also a good all-over body stretch that helps relieve fatigue and relaxes the neck. The walkback stretches the spine, hips, and hamstrings and tones the abdominals and internal organs. Use yoga breathing.

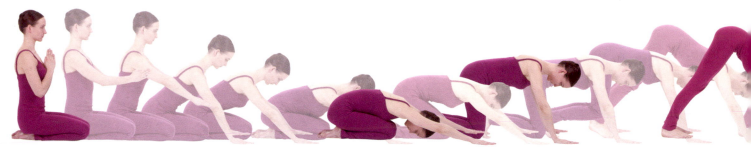

● Continue from the position on the previous page.

● Fold forward as you exhale, extending your arms. Spread your palms and hands into the floor. Your tummy and chest should rest on top of your thighs.

● Move onto all fours as you inhale, moving your feet hip-width apart. Extend through the crown of your head and your tailbone, your shoulders drawing down your back and your shoulder blades drawing into your spine. Keep your neck long.

● As you exhale, tuck your toes under; then lift your hips high to come into the downward facing dog, straightening your legs and extending your heels and head down. Also keep your shoulders wide and your chest open. Hold for three to five breaths.

▶   **exhale**   ▶   **inhale**   ▶   **exhale**   ❚❚ ▶

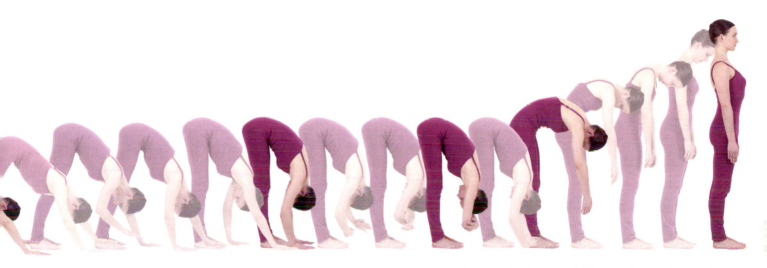

● Walk your hands back toward your feet as you inhale. Keep your head heavy and your pelvic floor and abdominals lifting.

● Once your hands have reached your feet, exhale as you bring each hand to the opposite elbow. Keep your legs strong and drawn up (you can bend them to lessen the intensity of the stretch). Hold for three to five breaths.

● Inhale as you release your hands and arms. Bend your knees and draw your tailbone down, lift your abdominals, and uncurl your body little by little, raising your head last.

● Bring your feet together, pressing them into the floor. Draw your leg muscles up and extend your tailbone down. Lift your abdomen, open your chest, and widen your shoulders. Keep your arms relaxed and neck long. Gaze forward. This is the mountain pose.

inhale ▶ exhale ❚❚ ▶ inhale ▶ exhale ❚❚

mighty pose into dancer balance

This is a vigorous upward stretch that tones the ankles and strengthens the leg muscles, spine, shoulders, and arms. It builds stamina, improves balance and stability, and enhances focus and concentration. This is a yoga breathing exercise.

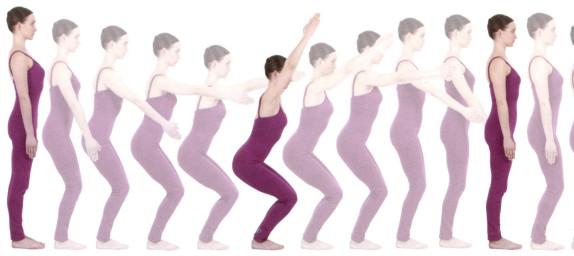

● Continue from the position on the previous page. As you exhale, bend your knees as if going to sit on a low stool. Stretch your arms above your head, palms facing inward, bringing your body into a zig-zag shape.

● Press your heels into the floor, squeezing your inner thighs together. Draw your abdominals in, lift your side ribs and armpits, and stretch your arms, keeping a long, easy neck. Hold the pose for five breaths.

● Come back up to standing as you inhale by lowering your arms and straightening your legs. Then breathe normally.

▶ **exhale**   ❚❚ ▶ **inhale and breathe normally**   ▶

● Standing tall, exhale as you bend your right knee, and bring your foot up behind you. Catch your foot with your right hand. Maintain a stable center.

● Inhale as you stretch your left arm above your head, palm facing inward. Press your left foot firmly into the floor, spreading your toes and drawing up your standing leg. Lift your pelvic floor and relax your neck and shoulders. Hold the balance for five breaths.

● With control, release the leg as you exhale, lower your left arm and go back into the standing position.

● Stand tall and easy in mountain pose, breathing normally. Then repeat on the left leg.

| exhale | ▶ | inhale | ⏸ ▶ | exhale | ▶ | breathe normally | ⏸ |

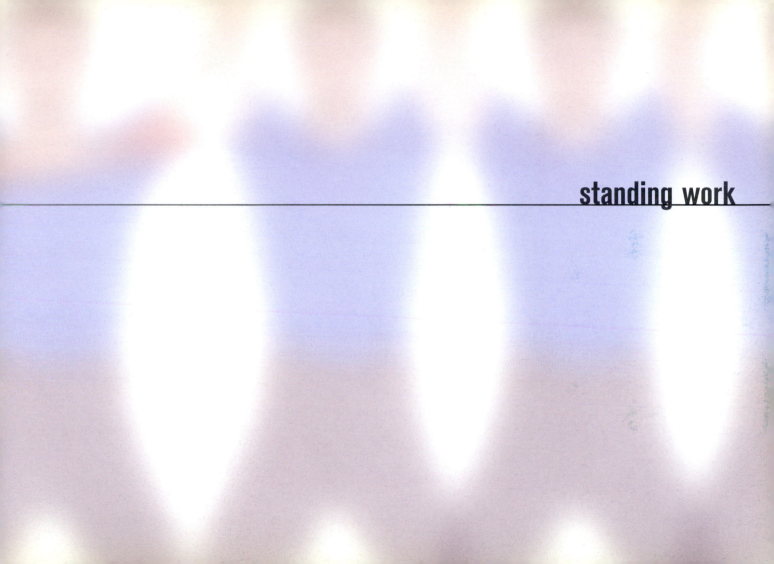

standing work

starter connecting movement

This movement starts every fusion sequence. The movement should flow with your breath while developing flexibility for the whole body. Use yoga breathing.

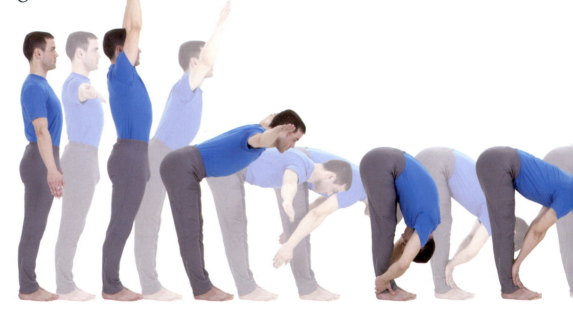

● Continue from the position on the previous page.

● As you inhale, lift your arms out to your sides and slowly turn the palms of your hands to face inward as you come into the full extension above your head.

● With feet and legs firm, squeeze your inner thighs together. As you exhale, start to bend forward, hinging from the hips and lowering your arms as your body comes down. Catch your ankles with your hands as your head folds in.

▶   **inhale**   ▶   **exhale**   ▶

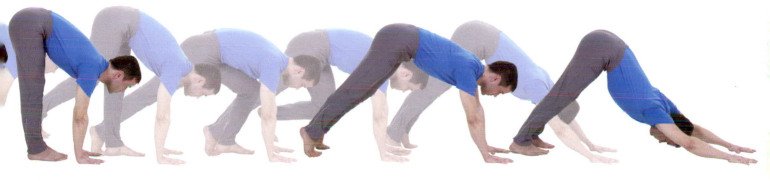

● Lift and lengthen your abdominals and place your hands on your shins. Lift your chin and chest, concave your spine, and extend your tailbone to the ceiling. Inhale as you do so.

● Still inhaling, place your hands on the floor (bending your knees if necessary), draw your abdominals up strongly, and then start to walk back, one leg at a time (or jump with both feet together).

● Land softly as you start to exhale, knees slightly bent and feet hip width apart.

● Still exhaling, stretch out your arms and legs, your hips high toward the ceiling, extending into the full downward dog position. Continue onto the ending movement on the next page.

inhale ▶ ▶ **exhale** ▶ ❚❚

ending movement

standing work

This flowing movement ends all fusion sequences. Beginners can join the starter connecting movement and the ending movement together to make their own dynamic exercise. Use yoga breathing.

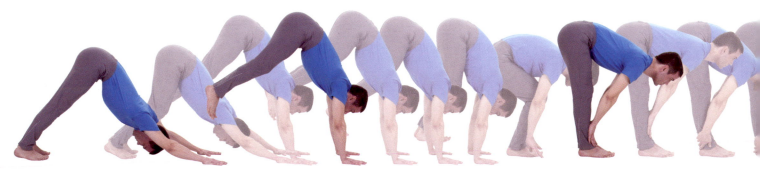

● Continue from the position on the previous page. Hold the downward dog pose for five breaths.

● Bend your knees and lift your hips higher toward the ceiling as you exhale. Draw your thigh muscles up, engage your pelvic floor, and draw your abdominals back strongly.

● As you inhale, spring from your toes and jump your feet forward to land in between your hands. Bend your knees as you land. Keep your hips pushed toward the ceiling and your hands pushed firmly into the floor as you do so. Jump with control.

● Still inhaling, continue the movement, placing your hands on your shins. Keep your chin and chest lifted and your spine concave. Avoid over-extending your neck.

▶　　　　　　　　　▶　　**exhale**　　　　▶　　**inhale**　　　　▶　　　　　　　　　▶

- Slide your hands down around the backs of your ankles as you fold your body against your legs, exhaling as you do so. To ease the intensity of the stretch, bend your knees slightly.

- With your feet and legs firm, inhale as you start to lift your chest, hinging from the hips. Lead with your heart as you come up, letting your arms float up to the side.

- Come up to standing as you continue to inhale, drawing your tailbone down and lifting your spine. Stretch your arms over your head and bring your palms together.

- Standing tall, exhale as you draw your shoulder blades down and let your palms come down through the center line of your body, finishing in prayer pose.

exhale ▶ inhale ▶ ▶ exhale ‖

fusion 1 *standing work*

Fusion 1 teaches you how to synchronize the movement of your arms and legs and encourages upper body strength. The lunges contained in the movement strengthen your legs and hips, and the twists relieve tension in the ribcage and spine. The sequence also tones and massages your internal organs. Use yoga breathing.

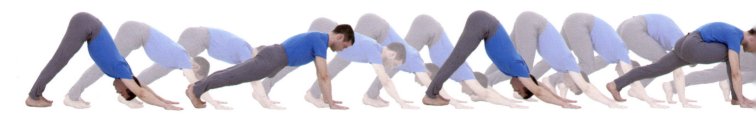

● Begin with the starter connecting movement (see pp. 44–45) to take you into the downward facing dog.

● Move your hips downward and forward as you inhale, so your body is long and flat like a plank. Extend through your legs and heels, spreading your palms and fingers into the floor. Keep your abdominals lifting to support your lower back.

● Lift your hips high and back into the downward facing dog pose as you exhale.

● With control, step your right foot forward between your hands, to the inside of your right hand. Inhale as you do so. Keep your back leg extended. Your right knee should be directly above your right foot.

■   **inhale** ▶   **exhale** ▶   **inhale** ▶

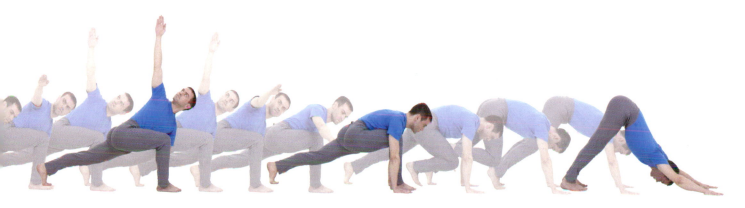

● As you exhale, move your left hand in underneath your left shoulder. Lift your right arm toward the ceiling, turning your abdomen and chest from your hips to follow your arm. Follow your hand with your eyes. Hold for two or three breaths.

● Come back down as you inhale, lowering your arm back down to the floor.

● With a strong abdominal lift, pressing your hands into the floor, move your right leg back and push your hips to the ceiling into the downward facing dog position. Exhale as you do so.

● Continue to exhale as you expand into the downward facing dog. Hold for three to five breaths; then repeat on the other leg, starting with the plank. Finish with the ending sequence (see pp. 46–47).

exhale   ❙❙ ▶   inhale   ▶   exhale   ▶   ❙❙

fusion 2

Fusion 2 also uses a lunge, which opens the groin and stretches the front of the thigh. Lifting the arms strengthens the back, shoulders, and arms. The movement also improves balance and stamina. Remember to keep breathing during the sequence, which is a yoga breathing exercise.

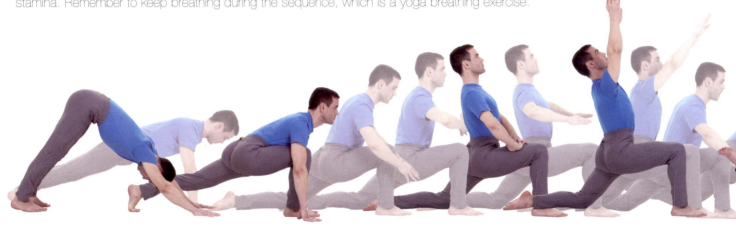

● Begin with the starter connecting movement (see pp. 44–45) to finish in a downward facing dog.

● Step forward as in Fusion 1 as you inhale.

● Exhale as you lower your left knee to the floor and lift your trunk. Extend your tailbone down and keep drawing your abdominals back. Then, as you inhale, bring your hands up, interlock your fingers, and press down on your right thigh.

● From a firm base, exhale as you lift your back and side ribs, open your chest, and extend your arms toward the ceiling, palms facing each other. Remember to keep breathing. Hold for three to five breaths.

| ■ | inhale | ▶ | exhale and inhale | ▶ | exhale | ‖ ▶ |

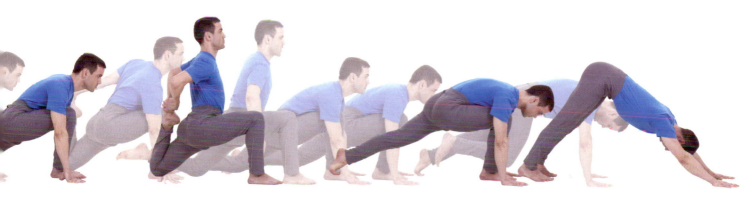

● Come back down as you inhale and place your hands back on the floor either side of your right foot, sliding your left knee back slightly and pulling your left foot off the floor.

● From a strong center, lift your chest. As you exhale, place your hands behind you, one at a time, and catch your left foot. Keep your trunk lifting as you pull your heel in toward your buttock. Keep your right leg strong. Hold for three to five breaths.

● Release your left foot and, as you inhale, place both hands back on the floor, tucking the toes of your left foot under.

● Lift your hips high and, as you exhale, step your right foot back, extending your spine to the downward facing dog position. Repeat on the left leg; then finish with the ending movement (see pp. 46–47).

inhale ▶ exhale ❚❚ ▶ inhale ▶ exhale ❚❚

fusion 3 *standing work*

Fusion 3 is a good sequence for strengthening both the upper and lower body.

It particularly strengthens the wrists, waist, chest, and arms. Use yoga breathing.

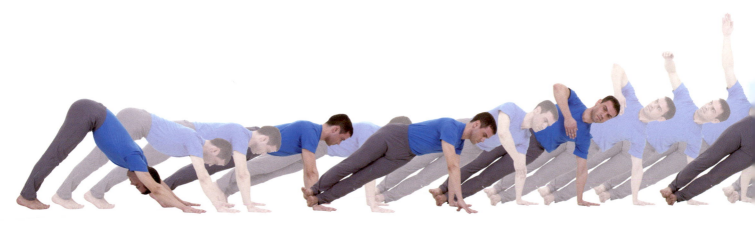

● Begin with the starter connecting movement to take you into the downward facing dog. Then exhale as you bring both feet together to form one "big" leg.

● As you inhale, squeeze your inner thighs together and bring your hips down into the plank.

● Keep extending strongly through your heels. As you exhale, stretch your legs fully and start to shift your weight onto your left hand and the outer edge of your left foot. Start to move your right hand off the floor.

● Push your left hip up through your right hip and push your right hip up to the ceiling, while continuing to turn side-on to the floor. Bring your right arm across your chest. Inhale as you do so.

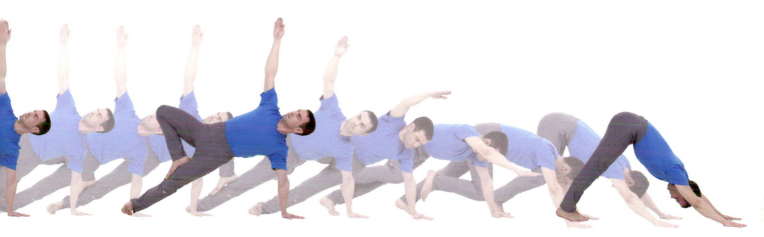

● Extend into the pose as you exhale, opening your chest and fully extending your arm to the ceiling. Press your left hand firmly into the floor, drawing the left arm up. Hold for three to five breaths.

● To increase the stretch, draw your right foot up the inside of your left leg. Keep your right hip lifted to the ceiling and your right leg strong. Hold for three to five breaths.

● To come out of the pose, curl your extended arm and upper body down with control and release your right leg. Inhale as you do so.

● As you exhale, place your right hand back on the floor, setting your feet back in the downward facing dog position. Repeat on the other side; then finish with the ending movement.

exhale inhale exhale

fusion 4—warrior sequence

Fusion 4 is an advanced sequence that generates all-over body strength and promotes dynamic movement. It will require all your focus and attention. This is a yoga breathing exercise.

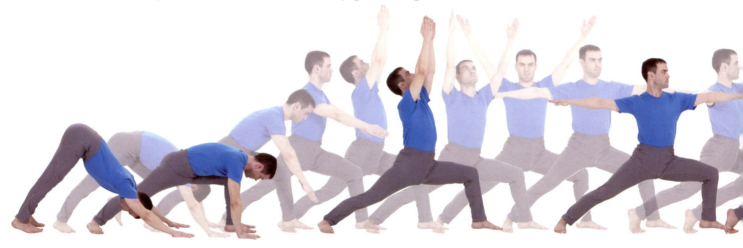

● Begin with the starter connecting movement to take you into the downward facing dog.

● Turn your right foot out at 45 degrees so the outer edge of your foot is pressed firmly into the floor. Then as you inhale, step your left foot forward between your hands, making sure your left knee is directly over your left ankle.

● Moving from a firm base and strong center, continue to inhale as you float your arms out to the side and up over your head. This brings you into Warrior 1. Keep your trunk lifted and your neck long and easy. Hold for three to five breaths.

● Turn your right foot out further and inhale as you draw your right hip back while pushing your left hip forward and turning your trunk. Move your arms down to shoulder height. Exhale as you turn your head. This is Warrior 2 pose. Hold for three to five breaths.

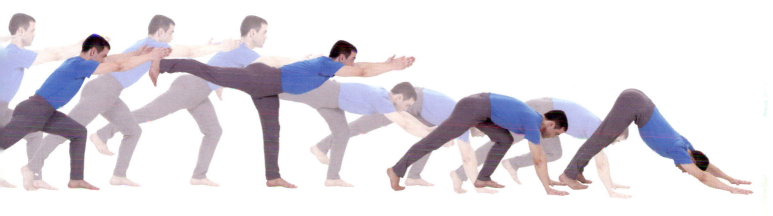

● Inhale as you turn your hips to face the direction of your left leg and bring your right heel off the floor. Your legs should be parallel. At the same time, move your right arm around to point in the same direction.

● Keeping your chin lifted, extend your trunk over your left thigh. Hop your right foot forward; then exhale as you push off the ground to raise your right leg. Shift your weight over your standing leg and extend. This is Warrior 3. Hold for three to five breaths.

● Bend your standing leg, and with control, place both hands on the floor, lowering your hips. Lower your right leg as you inhale.

● Push and extend your hips toward the ceiling as you exhale into a downward facing dog. Finish with the ending movement. Repeat the whole sequence on the other leg; then finish with the ending movement.

inhale ▶   exhale ⏸ ▶   inhale ▶   exhale ⏸

fusion 5

standing work

Fusion 5 strengthens the leg and back muscles and loosens the hips. The extended swan contained in this movement brings a deep stretch to the hips and buttocks. Use yoga breathing.

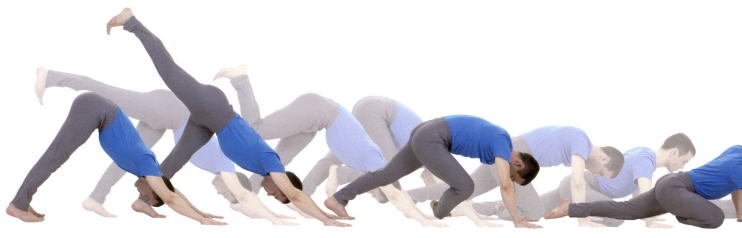

● Begin with your starter connecting movement to take you into the downward facing dog.

● As you inhale, release your right leg up to the ceiling. Hold and exhale. Press your hands and left foot firmly into the floor as you extend your right leg.

● Bend your right knee as you inhale; then lower your hips and start to swing your right leg through.

● Gazing ahead and still inhaling, lower your right knee by your right hand. Tuck your right foot under your left hip and slide your left leg back.

■   inhale and exhale   ❚❚ ▶   inhale   ▶   ▶

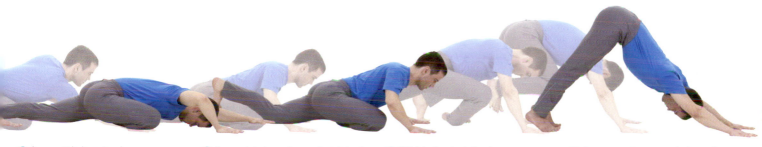

● As you exhale, extend your arms and body forward over your right leg and place your forehead on the floor. Sink into the floor and relax. Hold for five breaths.

● As you inhale, walk your hands back to lift up your body.

● Still inhaling, tuck the toes on your left foot under. Keep your chest lifted and gaze ahead.

● As you continue to exhale, push your hands into the floor and, moving from a strong center, lift your hips high to the ceiling. Set your feet and come up into the downward facing dog. Repeat on the other leg; then finish with the ending movement.

  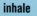

advanced connecting move

Add this advanced set of movements to the end of any fusion sequence before you do your ending movement sequence. This produces a strong dynamic routine. This sequence introduces the crocodile and the upward facing dog. Use yoga breathing.

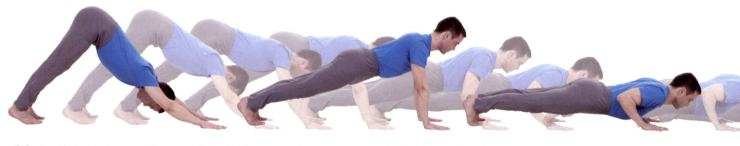

● Begin with the starter connecting movement to end in the downward facing dog.

● Start to lower your hips as you inhale and come down into the plank.

● Extend through your legs and push your heels back.

● As you exhale, lower your body to 2in (5cm) above the ground, gazing ahead. Bend your arms, keeping them against your sides and draw your shoulders down. This is the crocodile position.

■   **inhale**   ▶   ▶   **exhale**   ▶

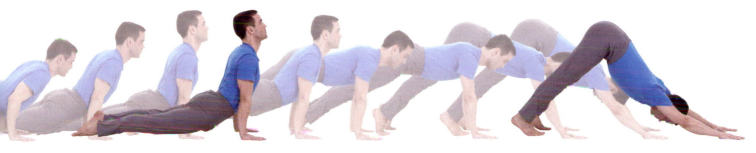

● Keeping a strong lift in your abdominals, inhale as you roll over your toes so the tops of your feet are flat on the floor.

● Straighten your arms as you lift the front of your hips, your body still off the floor. Lengthen and lift the whole of your spine, opening your chest. Inhale as you do so.

● Coming from a strong center, exhale as you push your hands into the floor, roll back over your toes, and lift your hips up to the ceiling.

● Set your feet and legs as you expand into a downward facing dog. Hold for five breaths; then finish with the ending movement.

inhale ▶ **inhale** ▶ **exhale** ▶ ‖

the eagle
standing work

This entwining balance exercise strengthens the legs, stretches the arms and shoulder blades, and improves focus and concentration. This is a yoga breathing exercise.

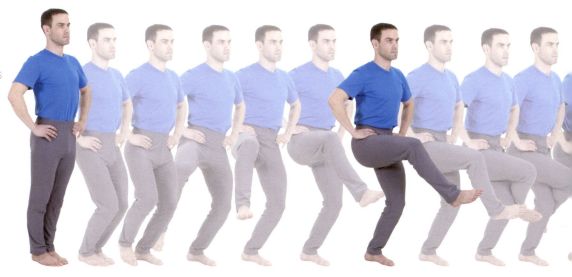

● Stand tall with your hands on your hips, gazing straight ahead.

● Inhale as you press your feet into the floor and bend your knees. Lift and extend your trunk.

● Exhale as you start to swing your right leg out to the side, and bending your right knee, cross it over your left leg. Keep a strong center.

inhale ▶ exhale ▶

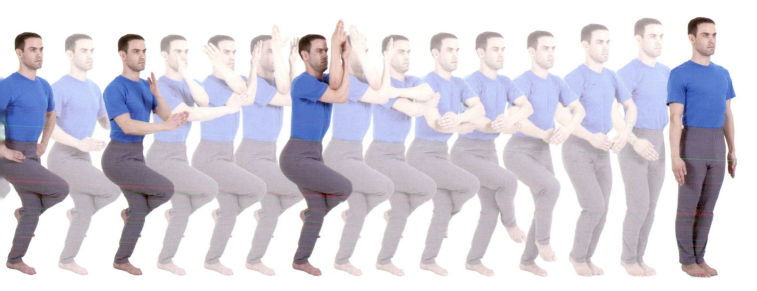

● While maintaining your balance, tuck the toes on your right foot behind your left calf, taking your hands off your hips. Keep spreading and pressing your standing foot into the floor. Inhale as you do so.

● With your elbows bent, exhale as you cross your left elbow over your right with your forearms stretching to the ceiling, your thumbs facing your head, and the palms of your hands together. Hold for five breaths, lifting and extending your trunk.

● Release your arms and legs at the same time as you exhale.

● Finish by standing tall; then repeat on the other leg. With practice, you will gradually learn to synchronize the movements of your arms and legs.

inhale ▶   exhale ❚❚ ▶   exhale ▶   ❚❚

palm tree 1

This side movement exercises, stretches, and tones the waist, upper back, and spine.

This is a pilates breathing exercise.

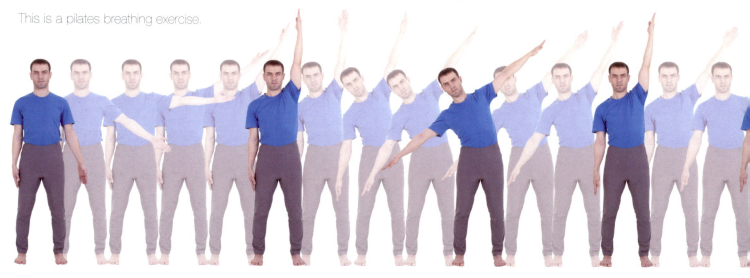

● Stand tall with your feet hip width apart.

● As you inhale, raise your left arm out to the side and up over your head, palm facing in.

● Keeping your shoulder blades down, start to dip to the right as you exhale, bending from the waist. Raise your right arm until your shoulders and arms are in a diagonal line like wings, palms facing downward.

● As you inhale, lower your right arm down to your side and lift and turn your left arm back up over your head. Come back up to upright, your palms facing inward as before.

| ■ | **inhale** ▶ | **exhale** ▶ | **inhale** ▶ |

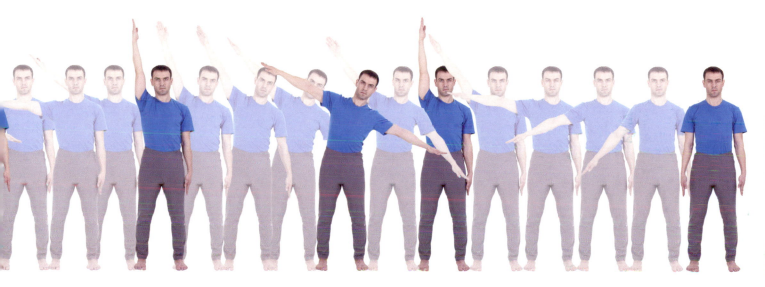

● Lower your left arm down to your side as you exhale.

● Lift your right arm up to the ceiling as you inhale, palms facing inward. Remember to keep your hips and shoulders facing the front.

● Dip to the left as you exhale, raising your left arm so your arms are in a diagonal line, palms facing down. Then as you inhale, lower your left arm and lift and turn your right arm back up over your head, coming back to an upright position, palms facing inward.

● Exhale as you lower your right arm down to your side, keeping your trunk lifted. Finish with normal, easy breathing.

exhale ▶ **inhale** ▶ **exhale and inhale** ▶ **exhale** ‖

palm tree 2

This flowing sequence works on and stretches the wrists, arms, fingers, upper and lower back, and chest. It also tones the waist and improves shoulder flexibility. Use yoga breathing.

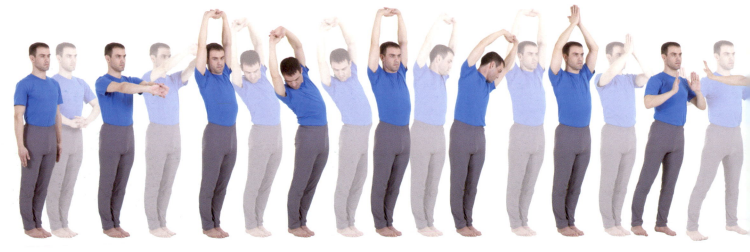

● Stand tall in mountain pose. Inhale as you interlock your fingers, push your palms away, and stretch your arms up over your head. Keep lengthening your abdomen.

● Exhale as you turn your head to look down at your right foot, bending at the waist. Extend through your arms; then from a strong center, come back to an upright position as you inhale. Repeat to the left.

● As you exhale, place the palms of your hands together in the prayer pose and draw them down the center line of your body, bringing your thumbs to rest on your sternum. Inhale and pause.

● As you exhale, step out to the side with your right foot so your feet are hip's width apart. With a strong action, push and spread the palms of your hands away from you. Inhale and pause, lifting and lengthening your abdominals.

▶   **exhale and inhale**   ❚❚ ▶   **exhale and inhale**   ❚❚ ▶   **exhale and inhale**   ❚❚ ▶

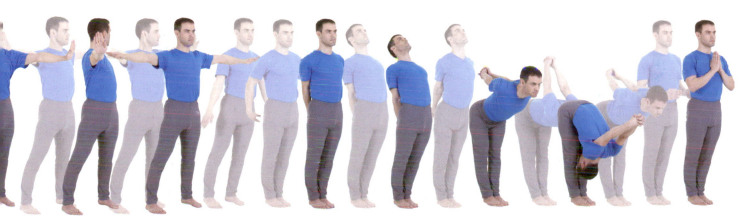

● Exhale as you turn from the waist to the right to look at your right hand. Keep your hips facing the front. Inhale as you come back to the center. Repeat to the left and come back to the center.

● Interlock your fingers behind your back and slide your feet together as you exhale. Pull your hands and tailbone down, lifting and opening your chest to the ceiling as you inhale.

● As you exhale, come into a forward bend, leading with your heart and bending from the hips. Take your arms up and over your head. Hold for five breaths, keeping a firm base and a strong center. Your head should be heavy.

● Lifting your pelvic floor and abdominals, inhale as you draw your tailbone down and come back to upright, bringing your hands into the prayer pose.

exhale and inhale   **exhale and inhale**    **exhale**   **inhale**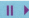

moving horse *standing work*

The moving horse strengthens your legs and improves coordination between your arms and legs. It also develops balance and tones the inner thighs, buttocks, calves, and feet. This is a pilates breathing exercise.

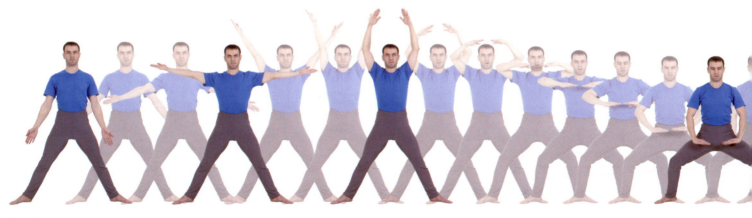

● Stand tall with your feet and legs turned out from your hips. Your arms should be by your sides, palms facing forward. Gaze straight ahead.

● As you inhale, strongly lift your arms up over your head, palms turning upward.

● Keep lifting your trunk and drawing your tailbone down and in. Also, keep lifting your pelvic floor and drawing your abdominals in.

● As you exhale, bend your knees slowly and press your knees and thighs back, moving your hands down as if your palms are pressing down on the air. Your hands should finish just below your navel.

■   **inhale**   ▶   ▶   **exhale**   ▶

● As you inhale, press your feet down, straighten your legs, and lift your arms back over your head with your palms facing in. Repeat this sequence four times. Finish with the palms of your hands together over your head.

● Exhale as you draw your hands down through the center line of your body, finishing with your thumbs in front of your sternum in prayer pose. Hold for five breaths.

● Keep your feet and legs firm, your center strong, and your chest open. Also keep your shoulders relaxed and wide and your neck long and easy. Gaze straight ahead.

● Inhale as you release your hands and straighten your legs as you come back to the starting position. Breathe normally.

inhale ❚❚ ▶ exhale ❚❚ ▶ ▶ inhale and breathe normally ❚❚

wide standing bend

The wide standing forward bend is a resting pose that improves flexibility in the hips, hamstrings, and spine. It also tones the internal organs, bringing circulation to the kidneys. Use yoga breathing.

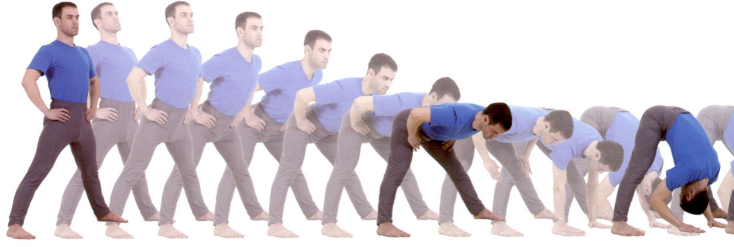

● Place your feet about 4½ft (1.5m) apart, and hands on your hips. Press your feet into the ground, drawing your legs up and opening your chest. Inhale.

● As you exhale, hinge forward from your hips keeping your trunk long, your back wide and strong, and your abdomen lifted.

● Extend through the crown of your head and your tailbone, keeping your neck long.

● Lower your arms to the floor, spreading your hands and fingers into the ground as you let the weight of your head take your body down. Keep drawing your inner ankles, inner thighs, and pelvic floor up.

■ inhale   exhale   ▶   ▶   ▶

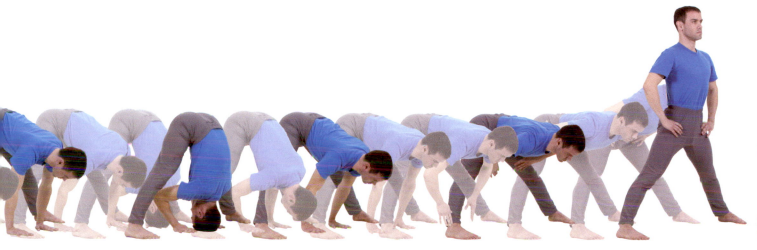

● Coming from a strong center, lift your chin and chest, concaving your spine. Also lift and lengthen your abdominals. Inhale as you do so.

● As you exhale, walk your hands back between your legs, shoulder width apart and elbows pointing straight back. Bring the crown of your head toward the floor. Bend your knees if you need to lessen the stretch. Hold for five breaths.

● From a strong center, inhale as you lift your chin and chest back up, extending your spine. Then as you exhale, press your feet firmly into the floor, drawing up through your legs. Place your hands on your hips.

● Hinge from your hips as you lift your body back to standing. Inhale as you do so.

inhale ▶ exhale ‖ ▶ inhale and exhale ▶ inhale ‖

arm release

The twisting arm action in this exercise increases circulation to the spine, keeping it supple.

Use yoga breathing.

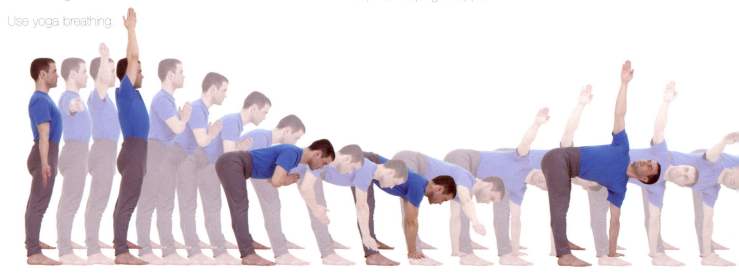

● Continue from the position on the previous page, your feet firm, legs drawing up, and your trunk lifted. Gaze straight ahead. Then as you inhale, stretch your arms up above your head, bringing your palms together.

● As you exhale, bring your palms down to prayer pose. Hinge forward from your hips, keeping your back long and chest lifted.

● Bring your trunk down, lowering your hands onto the floor. Keep the heels of your hands together, palms and fingers spreading and pointing to the side. Also keep your waist long and your chest lifting.

● As you inhale, lift your right arm up toward the ceiling, turning your trunk from the waist. Follow your arm with your eyes. Then as you exhale, bring your hand back down to the starting position. Repeat on the other side. Do two more sets on each side.

exhale ▶ **inhale and exhale** ❚❚ ▶

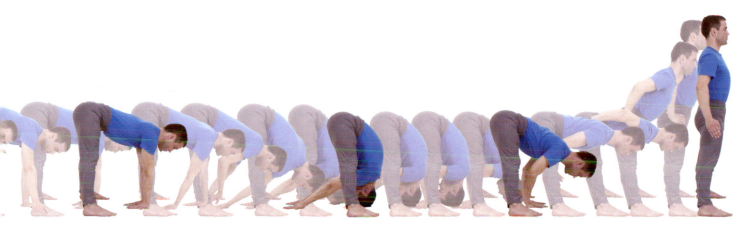

● As you inhale, turn your hands so that your fingers point backward between your legs. Keep your trunk long and lifted.

● Keeping your feet and legs strong and your abdominals lifted, start to walk your hands through your legs, bringing your body down. Take your head, shoulders, and chest through, exhaling as you do so. Hold for three to five breaths.

● As you inhale, walk your hands forward again while extending your trunk and lifting your chest. Turn your fingers to point forward.

● From a firm base and strong center, exhale as you place your hands on your hips. Inhale as you come back up to standing, keeping your back long and flat. As you exhale, release your arms down to your sides.

inhale ▶ **exhale** ❚❚ ▶ **inhale** ▶ **exhale, inhale, exhale** ❚❚

garland with rise

standing work

This exercise increases mobility in your pelvis and hip joints. It also relaxes and lengthens your back and buttock muscles and strengthens your feet, ankles, and calves. Use yoga breathing.

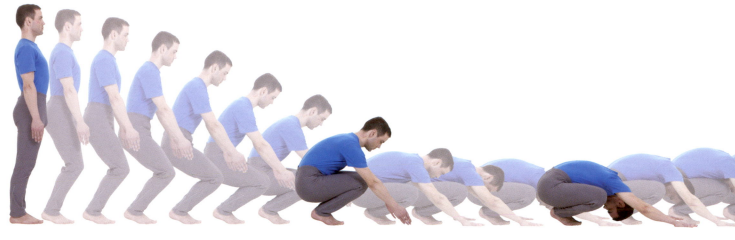

● Start by standing in mountain pose, with your abdomen lifted, your chest open, and your shoulders wide.

● With control, start to bend your knees and release your heels off the floor, inhaling as you do so. Start to lower your hips down to your heels, keeping your trunk lifted. Place your hands on the floor for support.

● Exhale as you extend your arms forward, spreading your palms and fingers into the floor. Keep your feet together and open your knees out to the sides.

● Feel the weight of your hips dropping toward your heels. Let your chest move down toward the floor and keep your head heavy and your neck long. Hold for five breaths.

▶ **inhale** ▶ **exhale** ▶ ❚❚ ▶

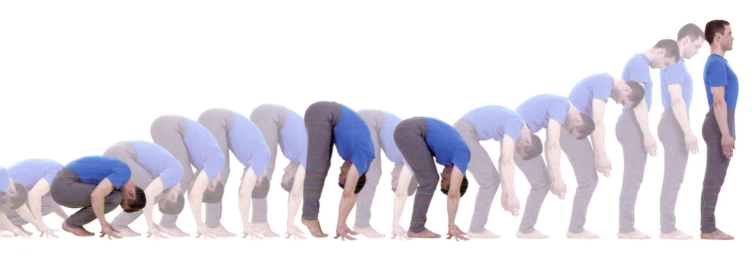

● Inhale as you bring your knees to meet each other, squeezing your thighs together. Walk your hands back, cupping them so only your fingertips touch the ground. Press the balls of your feet into the floor.

● Exhale as you straighten your legs, staying on the balls of your feet. Keep your abdominals lifting and let your head hang.

● Inhale as you press your heels back down into the floor, bending your knees.

● Still inhaling, bring your hands off the floor and come up to standing, uncurling gradually from your center. Finish in mountain pose.

inhale ▶ exhale ▶ inhale ▶ ❚❚

triangle *standing work*

The triangle stretches the sides of the spine, legs, and hips. This pose also stretches the muscles in between the ribs, opening the chest and encouraging deeper breathing. Use yoga breathing.

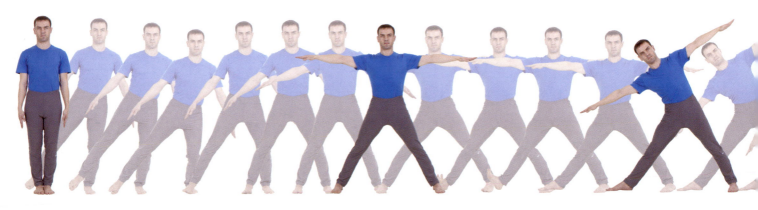

- Start in mountain pose, with your abdomen lifted, your chest open, and your shoulders wide.

- Soften your knees and start to step or spring out to the side, exhaling as you do so.

- Your feet should finish 4¹/₂ft (1.5m) apart. Lift and extend your arms out to shoulder height, your palms facing downward.

- As you inhale, turn your left foot in slightly and your right foot out to 90 degrees. Drawing your legs up and keeping your trunk lifted, hinge and extend from your hips, your arms held out like wings.

exhale ▶ ▶ **inhale** ▶

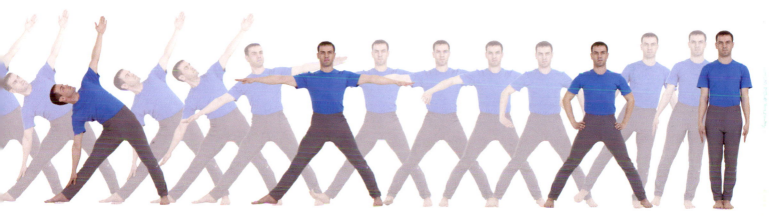

● As you exhale, place your right hand on your right shin, turning your head to the ceiling. Keep the outer edge of your left foot firm, your left hip turned up and back, and your right hip pressing forward. Extend through your left arm.

● With control, from a firm base and strong center, come back up to standing, inhaling as you do so. Repeat to the left.

● Still inhaling, turn your feet and legs to face forward, your hands on your hips.

● As you exhale, step or spring your feet back to mountain pose, lowering your arms to your sides.

exhale ▶ inhale ▶ ▶ exhale ❚❚

intense side stretch*work*

This sequence stretches your inner thigh and groin and strengthens your leg and buttock muscles. It also tones the waist and is a good stretch for the ribcage, encouraging deeper breathing. This is a yoga breathing exercise.

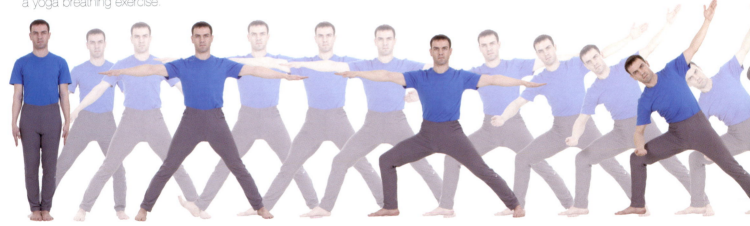

● Start in mountain pose, with your abdomen lifted, your chest open, and your shoulders wide.

● As you exhale, step or jump your feet 4¹/₂ft (1.5m) apart and release your arms up to shoulder height.

● Moving from a firm base and a strong center, inhale and turn your left foot in slightly and your right foot out to 90 degrees. Bend your right knee, which should be directly over your right ankle.

● Press firmly against the outer edge of your left foot as you exhale, drawing your right inner thigh up and back. Hinge from your hips and lower your right forearm to the top of your thigh. Start to release your left arm upward.

▶   **exhale**   ▶   **inhale**   ▶   **exhale**   ▶

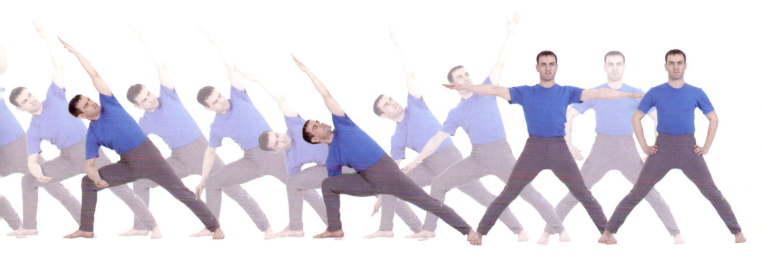

● Keep exhaling and extend your left arm up and over your head. Turn and look past your upper arm at the ceiling, keeping your chin down. Hold for three to five breaths.

● If you wish to take the stretch further, create a 90-degree angle at your knee by lowering your hips further and dropping your right hand to the floor behind your right ankle. Hold for three to five breaths.

● From a firm base and strong center, come back up to standing, inhaling as you do so. Keep your arms at shoulder height. Then repeat on the left side.

● As you exhale, lower your hands to your hips. Step or jump your feet together and come into mountain pose.

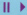 **inhale** **exhale and breathe normally**

turning intense stretch

You will need strong legs and hips for this pose, which improves flexibility in the spine. It also exercises your kidneys and abdominal organs, which aids digestion. Use yoga breathing.

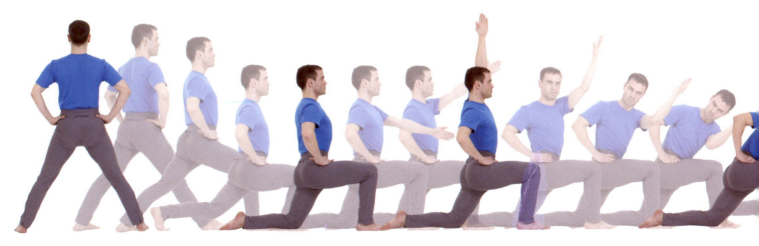

● Start in mountain pose; then exhale as you step or jump your feet wide apart.

● As you inhale, turn your feet, legs, and hips to the right, turning your trunk to come over your right leg. Keep your tailbone down and your sacrum in. As you exhale, lower your left knee down to the floor to come into a kneeling position.

● Extend your left arm up over your head as you inhale, your palm facing inward.

● Take your left elbow to the outer edge of your right thigh, turning the whole of your trunk around to follow it. Exhale as you do so.

▶ **exhale**　　　**inhale and exhale**　▶　**inhale**　　　▶　**exhale**　　▶

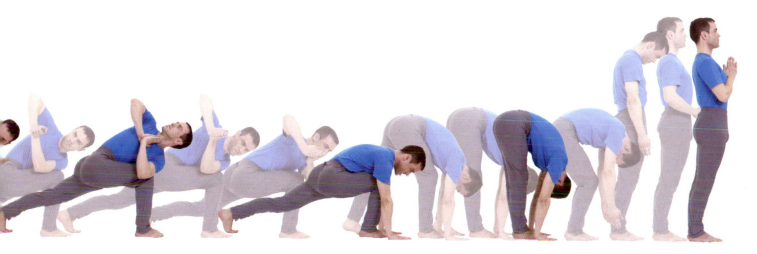

● Tuck the toes of your left foot under and, with a strong action, lift your left knee off the floor, extending strongly through your left leg and heel. Bring your hands into prayer pose, your elbows pointing at the floor and ceiling. Hold for five breaths.

● Release from the pose as you inhale, placing both hands on the floor to come into a lunge.

● Step your left foot forward to join the right as you exhale and come into a forward bend. Squeeze your legs together.

● Come up to mountain pose, your hands in prayer pose, inhaling as you gradually uncurl upward. Repeat on the other side.

‖ ▶ **inhale** ▶ **exhale** ▶ **inhale** ‖

standing forward bend

This sequence loosens stiff legs and hips. It tones the abdominals and lengthens and releases tension in the neck. This is a yoga breathing exercise.

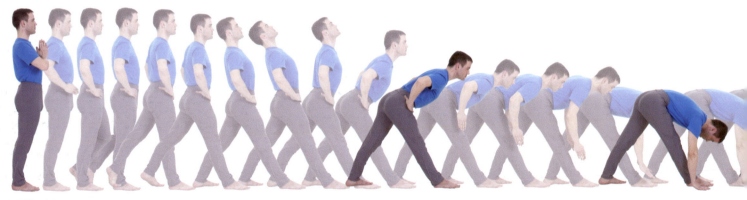

● Start in mountain pose, hands in prayer pose. As you exhale, step your left foot back by about 3ft (1m) and turn your left foot out at 45 degrees. Your right heel should be in line with your left instep, hips, and trunk facing forward.

● Press into the outer edge of your left foot, drawing your tailbone down, your sacrum in, and your back ribs up and in. Keep your chest open and your face to the ceiling. Inhale.

● Push firmly into your left heel and as you exhale, hinge downward from your hips, keeping your body long.

● Still exhaling, place your hands on the floor and relax your shoulders and neck. Then as you inhale, lift your chin and chest, extending through the crown of your head.

▶ **exhale**   ▶ **inhale**   ▶ **exhale**   ▶ **exhale and inhale**   ▶

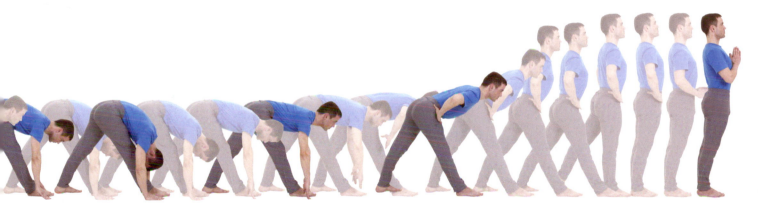

● Exhale and deepen into the pose, moving your chest down over your right leg.

● As you inhale, press firmly into your left heel, lifting and extending your trunk to concave your spine.

● From a firm base and strong center, place your hands on your hips as you exhale.

● Inhale as you come up to mountain pose by stepping your left foot forward to join your right, keeping your back lengthened. Pause and repeat on the other leg.

exhale　▶　inhale　▶　exhale　▶　inhale　‖

half moon balance

The half moon balance improves balance, coordination, and muscular stamina in your legs.

This is a yoga breathing exercise.

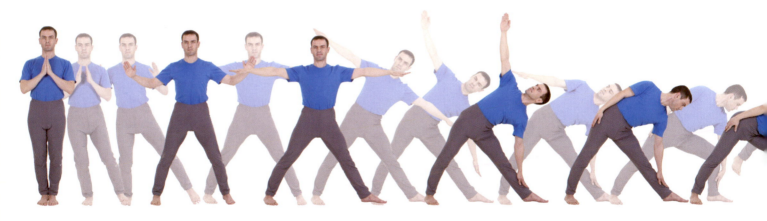

- Start in mountain pose, hands in prayer pose. Jump your feet 4ft (1.25m) apart as you exhale, extending your arms out to shoulder height.

- Turn your right foot in slightly, your left foot out at 90 degrees, and line your left heel up with your right instep. Inhale as you do so, drawing your legs up.

- Come into triangle pose (see pp. 74–75) as you exhale. Hinging from your hips, place your left hand on your left shin and extend your right hand up to the ceiling. Gaze upward toward it.

- Lower your right arm down to the side of your body and turn your head to look at your left foot. Bend your left leg and extend your left hand to the floor, 12in (30cm) in front of your little toe.

▶ **exhale**   ▶ **inhale**   ▶ **exhale**   ▶

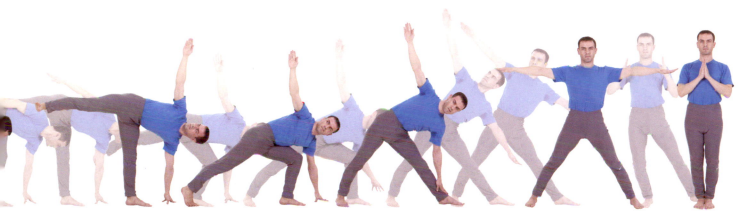

● Hop your right leg in toward your left heel as you inhale. Lift your right leg and hold it parallel to the floor. Then lift your right arm up to the ceiling, keeping your standing leg strong and extending through your lifted leg. Hold for three to five breaths.

● With control, bend your left leg as you exhale and lower your right leg to the ground.

● Still exhaling, come back into triangle pose.

● Come back up to standing as you inhale, turning your feet and legs to face the front. Then step or spring back to mountain pose as you exhale. Repeat on the other side.

inhale ❚❚ ▶   **exhale** ▶   ▶ **inhale and exhale** ❚❚

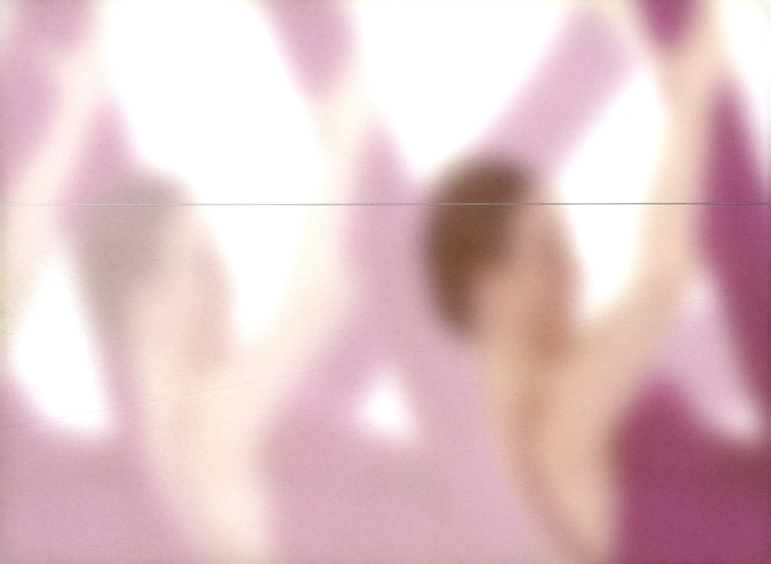

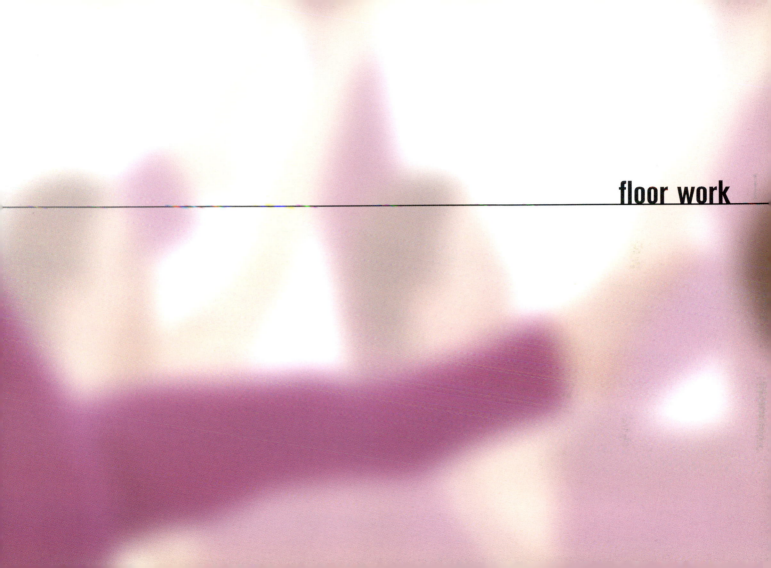

floor work

floor work

moving to the floor

This is a flowing sequence designed to bring you from standing work to floor work. As you start

to work on the floor, remember to move from a strong center with your neck held long and easy.

It is a pilates breathing movement.

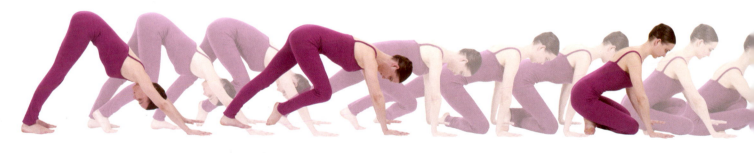

● Begin with the starter connecting movement to take you into the downward facing dog. Exhale.

● Bend your right knee and start to bring it forward as you inhale. Also start to lower your hips.

● Still inhaling, place your right shin on the floor, keeping your trunk extended upward.

● Still inhaling, draw your left leg in, crossing your ankles underneath you.

■ **exhale**　　　　　**inhale** ▶　　　　　▶　　　　　▶

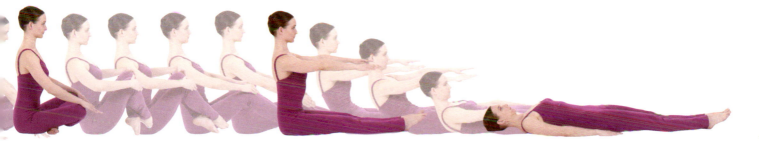

● Roll back into easy sitting pose as you exhale, your hands resting on your knees.

● Moving from a strong center with a long, easy neck, start to stretch your legs out and extend your arms as you inhale.

● Still inhaling, sitting up straight, fully extend your legs, keeping your arms long and soft.

● Engage your buttock and thigh muscles, tuck your tailbone slightly under, and draw your abdominals in. Then, roll back gradually as you exhale to come into resting pose, your palms facing downward. Pause.

exhale ▶ **inhale** ▶ ❚❚ ▶ **exhale** ❚❚

peel off the floor

This exercise stretches and strengthens the spine and tones the abdominals. Move fluidly and use your abdominals when performing this sequence. Do not jerk your neck or shoulders when rolling up. This is a pilates breathing exercise.

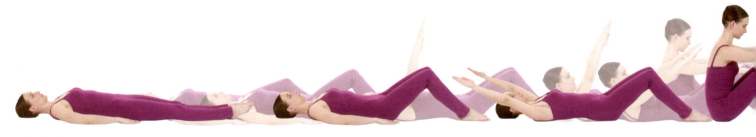

● Start by lying on your back in resting pose as before.

● Bring your knees up one at a time so your knees and feet are together. Press the soles of your feet firmly into the floor as you inhale.

● Exhale as you stretch your arms back over your head, finishing just above the floor. Draw your shoulder blades down your back and your abdominals in.

● Inhale as you bring your arms forward, your chin to your chest. Then exhale as you draw your abdominals in and peel your back off the floor, step by step. Curl forward up to sitting, your arms extended in front of you.

▶   **inhale**   ▶   **exhale**   ▶   **inhale and exhale**   ▶

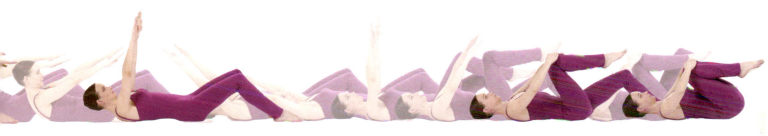

● Start to roll back down, inhaling as you squeeze your buttocks and slightly tuck your tailbone underneath you. Keep drawing your abdominals in.

● Exhale as you continue to roll down to the floor, step-by-step. Your head and shoulders should finish on the floor with your arms back over your head, slightly off the floor. Roll up and down four to eight times.

● Inhale as you bring one leg at a time up to your chest.

● Hug both knees to your chest; then exhale to release your lower back.

inhale ▶ **exhale** ❚❚ ▶ **inhale** ▶ **exhale** ❚❚

floor work

single leg abs

Single leg abs is an exercise that works your center, pelvic floor, and abdominals. As you work, remember to keep your hips and pelvis stable and your trunk anchored into the floor. It is a pilates breathing exercise.

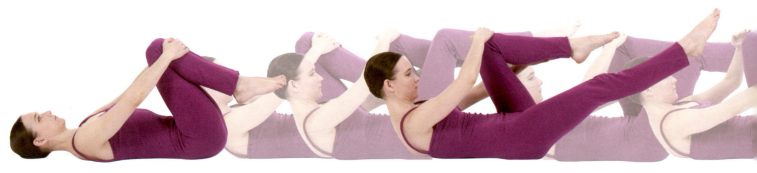

● Continue from the position on the previous page.

● As you exhale, take hold of your left leg and pull it to your chest, your right hand on your left knee and your left hand on your left calf, with elbows extending out. Keep your left shin parallel to the floor.

● Extend your right leg out in front of you, slightly higher than the level of your hips. Curl your head and shoulders off the floor.

● Inhale as you draw your abdominals in and slide your shoulders down your back.

▶ **exhale** ▶ ▶ **inhale** ▶

● Exhale as you swap legs and change your hands over. Keep your hips and pelvis stable and your trunk anchored into the floor. Change legs 10 to 20 times, inhaling for two leg changes, exhaling for the next two, and so on.

● If you have a weak back, extend your straight leg to the ceiling. This is easier than holding it at hip height.

● As you inhale, bring your legs together again, hugging them to your chest.

● Exhale as you lower your head and shoulders back down to the floor.

exhale   ❙❙ ▶   ▶   inhale   ▶   exhale   ❙❙

leg switch

The leg switch works the abdominals and the center body. It also loosens the hips and

stretches the backs of the legs. This is pilates breathing exercise.

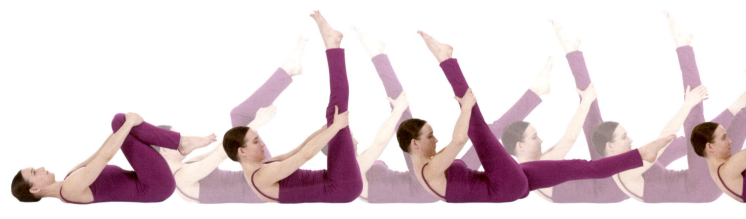

● Continue from the position on the previous page.

● As you exhale, stretch both legs to the ceiling as you draw your abdominals down. Place your hands on the backs of your thighs (or tops of your calves), anchoring your torso into the floor and lifting your head above your chest.

● As you inhale, lower your left leg to just above hip level, pulling your right leg in toward you, keeping it straight.

● As you exhale, quickly switch legs with rhythm and control.

▶   **exhale**   ▶   **inhale**   ▶   **exhale**   ▶

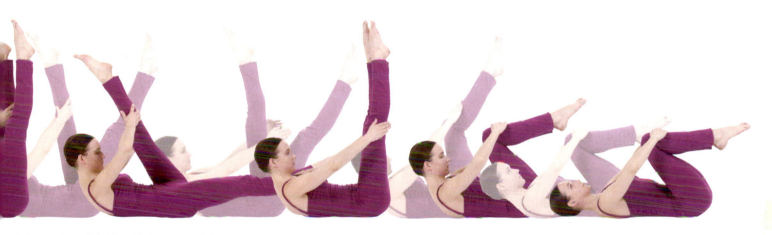

● Repeat the switch 10 to 20 times. Inhale for two switches; then exhale for two, and so on. Keep lifting your pelvic floor, drawing your abdominals in and looking down at your navel.

● To increase the intensity of the exercise, extend and hold your arms in front of you. Do not be tempted to catch your legs.

● Inhale as you bend your legs, catching your knees with your hands and pulling them toward your chest.

● Exhale as you lower your head and shoulders back to the floor.

double leg abs

This is a very strong abdominal exercise. Remember to keep your lower back flat against the floor as you raise and lower your legs. Also, remember to keep breathing. This is a pilates breathing exercise.

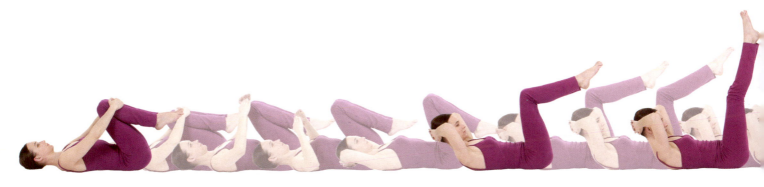

● Continue from the position on the previous page.

● As you inhale, place your hands behind your head, your elbows off the floor (so you can just see them out of the corner of your eye), and draw your abdominals in.

● Still inhaling, move your legs away from you and lift your feet so you have a right angle at your hips and knees.

● Exhale as you lift your head and shoulders off the floor, extending your legs to the ceiling.

inhale ▶ ▶ **exhale** ▶

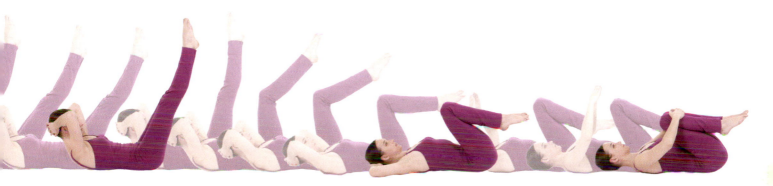

● As you inhale, lower your legs, keeping your trunk anchored into the ground. Do not lower your legs too far or you will lift your lower back off the floor, which must be avoided.

● Working from a strong center, bring your legs back up as you exhale.

● As you inhale, bend your legs and lower your head and shoulders to the floor. Repeat this exercise five to ten times.

● As you exhale, release your hands from behind your head and place them on your knees, pulling your knees to your chest. Rock slightly from side to side to massage your spine.

inhale ▶ exhale inhale ‖ ▶ exhale ‖

turn turn

Turn turn works the center body, waistline, and external obliques. It is important to remember to keep breathing as you turn from side to side. Also, do not pull on your neck with your hands— all the work should be done in the abdominal area. This is a pilates breathing exercise.

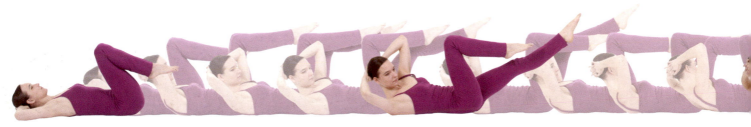

● Place your hands behind your head, elbows off the floor.

● Bring your head and shoulders off the floor as you exhale. Pause and, as you inhale, draw your abdominals in.

● As you exhale, extend your left leg, lifting and turning from your waist to the right. Bring your left elbow to your right knee, keeping your left shin parallel to the floor.

● Change legs as you inhale, keeping your elbows extended and your pelvis stable and level.

■   **exhale and inhale**   ▶   **exhale**   ▶   **inhale**   ▶

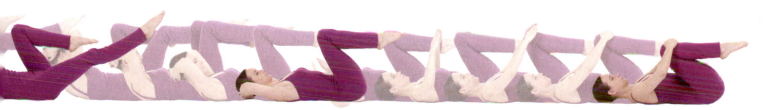

● Keep your extended leg lifted above hip height.

● Repeat 10 to 20 times, inhaling for two leg changes, then exhaling for the next two, and so on.

● Bring your knees together as you inhale.

● As you exhale, lower your head and shoulders to the floor, placing your hands on your shins.

▶ ‖ ▶ **inhale** ▶ **exhale** ‖

waist definer

This exercise tones and firms your waist and abdominals and massages your internal organs.

This is a pilates breathing exercise.

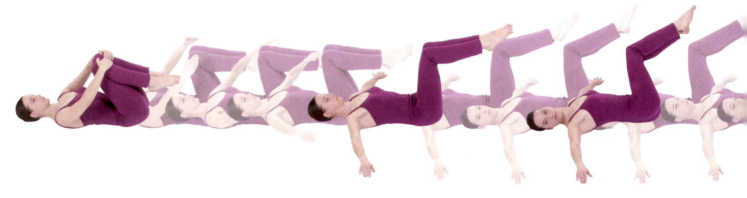

● Continue from the position on the previous page. Exhale as you hug your legs.

● Inhale as you release your arms and place them on the floor just below shoulder height. Keep your palms facing upward. For extra support, turn them to face downward.

● Move your legs away from you until they are at 90-degree angles at the hips and knees.

● Inhale as you squeeze your knees together, lifting your pelvic floor and drawing your abdominals in.

exhale   inhale   exhale   inhale

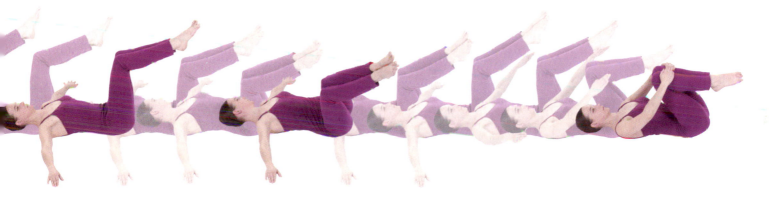

● With control, take your knees over to the left as you exhale, turning your head to the right. Keep your shoulders and upper back wide and flat against the floor. Avoid bringing your legs too low and keep your neck long.

● As you inhale, bring your legs and head back to center.

● As you exhale, take your legs over to the other side, moving your head in the opposite direction. As you inhale, come back to center. Repeat 10 to 20 times.

● Place your hands back on your knees and come back to the starting position. Exhale as you hug your knees.

exhale ▶ inhale ▶ exhale and inhale ❚❚ ▶ exhale ❚❚

floor work
waist and tummy stretch

The waist and tummy sequence stretches the ribs, waist, and hips. It brings relief to the lower back, but avoid this exercise if you have actual pain in your lower back or sacrum. Use yoga breathing.

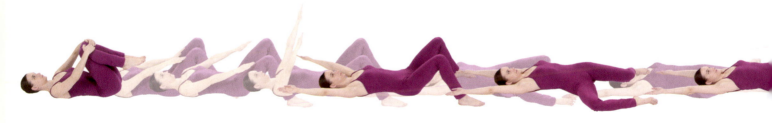

● Continue from the position on the previous page.

● As you exhale, place your feet flat on the floor more than hip's width apart. Extend your arms over your head.

● Inhale first; then as you exhale, bring both knees over to the right, taking the soles of your feet off the floor. Extend strongly through your left arm. Hold for five breaths, encouraging your breath to go into the left side of your ribs, waist, and hips.

● To intensify the stretch, place your right foot on your left knee while extending through your left arm. Hold for three to five breaths. With control, put your right foot back on the floor.

exhale ▶ **inhale and exhale** ❚❚ ▶ ❚❚ ▶

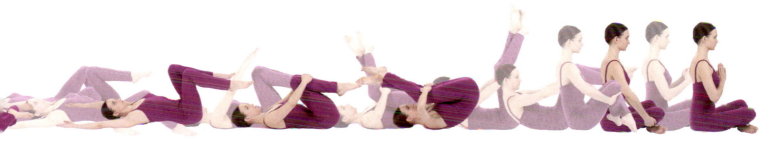

● As you inhale, extend through your tailbone and bring your knees back up to center. As you exhale, repeat on the other side, extending through your right arm.

● Exhale as you come back to center, placing your hands on the tops of your shins. Then cross your ankles, allowing your knees to move out to the side slightly. Place your hands behind your knees.

● Lift your pelvic floor and, with strong abdominals, inhale as you flick your feet over your head. Then with momentum, exhale as you roll back up to sitting.

● Bring your feet and legs back to easy pose, hands up to prayer pose and breathe normally.

inhale and exhale   ❚❚ ▶   **exhale**   ▶   **inhale and exhale**   ▶   **breathe normally**   ❚❚

floor work

basic back strengthener

This strong exercise strengthens and tones the buttocks, hamstrings, and back muscles. To make it easier, place a rolled-up towel under your thighs, but avoid this sequence if you have back problems. This is a yoga breathing exercise.

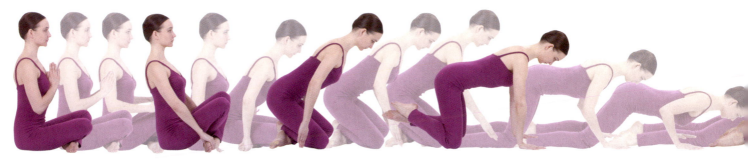

- Continue from the position on the previous page.

- Moving from a strong center, catch your feet as you inhale and pull them under your hips.

- Propel yourself forward as you exhale to come onto your hands and knees. Inhale and pause.

- Bending your elbows so your arms are parallel to your body, exhale as you lower your chest to the floor.

▶   **inhale**   ▶   **exhale and inhale**   ⏸ ▶   **exhale**   ▶

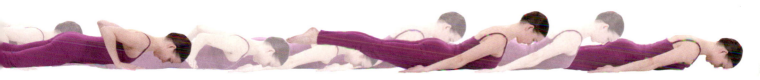

● Lying flat on the floor, extend your arms alongside your body, palms facing the ceiling.

● Inhale as you draw your shoulder blades down and extend your tailbone.

● Lift your head and legs off the floor as you exhale; then inhale as you expand into the pose, extending through your arms and legs. Keep lifting and lengthening your abdominals and keep your neck long and extended.

● Smoothly come back down as you exhale. Repeat three times.

▶ **inhale**   ▶ **exhale and inhale**   ▶ **exhale**   ‖

floor back lift *work*

The back lift stretches and strengthens all the muscles of the back, neck, and shoulders.
It also stretches the chest and abdomen, but avoid this exercise if you have back problems.
Also, remember not to throw your head back as you come up and use controlled movements
as you come back down. Use yoga breathing.

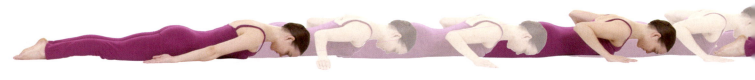

● Continue from the position on the previous page.

● Start to move your hands forward as you exhale.

● Place your hands on either side of your chest, fingertips under your shoulders.

● Inhale and spread the palms of your hands and fingers into the floor, your elbows pulling in toward your body. Keep extending through your legs and tailbone and keep your shoulders sliding down your back.

exhale ▶ ▶ **inhale** ▶

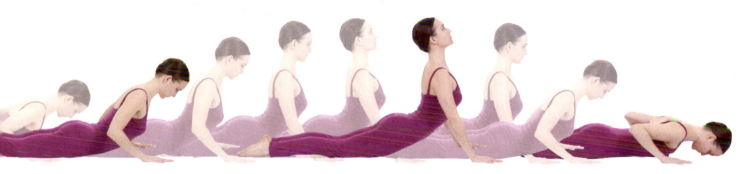

● Start to exhale as you push your hands into the floor and start to straighten your arms.

● Continue exhaling as you lift your head and chest off the floor and come up into a back bend. Fully straighten your arms, keeping your thighs and hips pressed into the floor.

● Lift and lengthen your abdominals, moving your back ribs in. Open and lift your chest, keeping your neck long and your chin slightly lifted (do not throw your head back). Hold for three to five breaths.

● With control, lower your body to its starting position as you exhale.

exhale ▶ ▶ ‖ ▶ exhale ‖

full back strengthener

The full back strengthener is a strong stretch for the shoulders, upper back, and fronts of the thighs. It is important to use controlled, smooth movements when doing this stretch. Do not jerk or strain. This is a yoga breathing exercise.

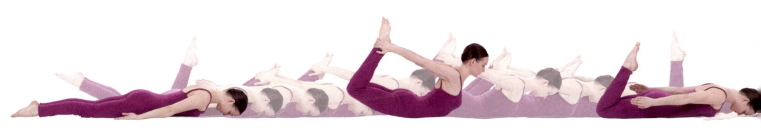

● Continue from the position on the previous page.

● Bend your knees and as you exhale, catch your ankles behind you. Inhale as you press your hips into the floor.

● As you exhale, lift your thighs and upper body off the floor, extending the crown of your head and your feet up toward the ceiling. Pull your feet away from your hands. Keep a long easy neck. Hold for five breaths.

● With control, release your feet and come back down to the floor. Exhale as you do so.

exhale and inhale ▶ exhale ❚❚ ▶ exhale ▶

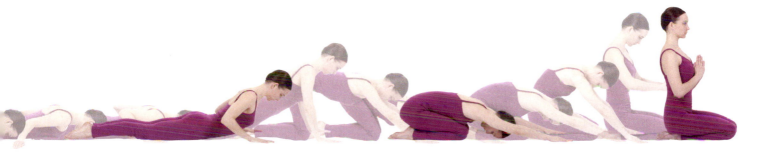

● As you inhale, extend your legs and place your hands on either side of your chest.

● Press your hands into the floor as you exhale and push your body upward, moving your hips back toward your heels, hinging at your hips and knees.

● Lower your tailbone and hips onto your heels and extend your arms forward, resting your forehead on the floor. Hold for three to five breaths.

● With your hips on your heels, slowly curl upward as you inhale, extending your spine and bringing your hands into prayer pose. Gaze straight ahead.

inhale ▶ exhale ▶ ❚❚ ▶ inhale ❚❚

intense spine stretch

This exercise is a powerful back bend that stretches and tones the whole spine. It also opens the chest, which helps encourage deeper breathing. Use yoga breathing.

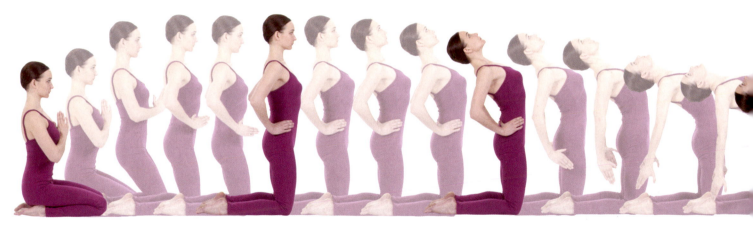

- Continue from the position on the previous page.

- Come up onto your knees as you inhale. Place your hands on your hips and press the tops of your feet and shins into the floor to create a firm base. Draw your thigh muscles up.

- As you exhale, draw your tailbone down, lift up through your hips, and open your chest to the ceiling. Pause and inhale.

- Keeping the lift in your chest, catch your heels or place your palms on the soles of your feet. Exhale as you do so.

▶ **inhale** ▶ **exhale and inhale** ‖ ▶ **exhale** ▶

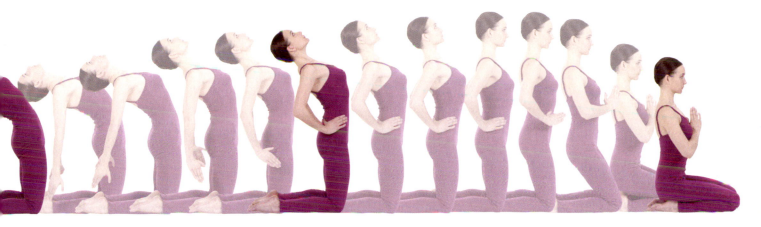

● While in the pose, keep your hips directly above your knees. Keep drawing your tailbone down and in. Hold for five breaths, your face relaxed.

● Moving from a strong center and a firm base, release your hands from your feet and come back up as you inhale.

● Place your hands on your hips and gaze ahead. Keep lifting through your hips and extending your trunk.

● Exhale as you lower your hips down onto your heels and bring your hands up to prayer pose. Hold for five to ten breaths.

inhale   exhale

child

floor work

This is a restful pose that brings relief to the back. It is the counter pose to the previous back bend exercises shown on pages 102–109. This is a yoga breathing exercise.

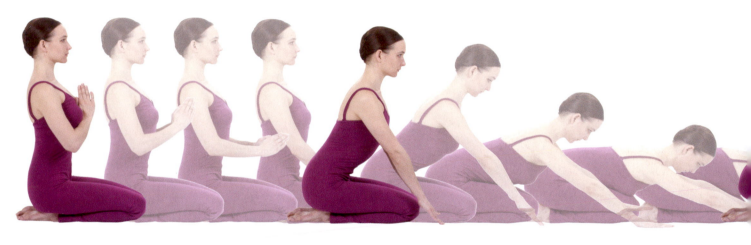

● Continue from the position on the previous page.

● As you inhale, place your hands on the floor, spreading your palms and fingers into the ground. Keep the weight of your hips dropping into your heels.

● Exhale as you slide your hands forward.

● Bring your tummy and chest to rest on the tops of your thighs.

▶ **inhale** ▶ **exhale** ▶ ▶

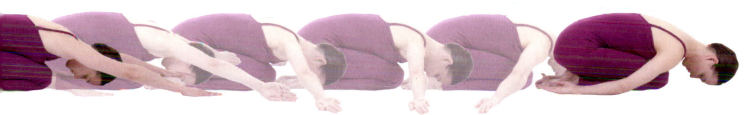

● Rest your forehead on the floor and keep your shoulder blades sliding down your back.

● If your head does not reach the floor, use a foam block or firm pillow to support your head.

● Keeping the extension in your arms, bring your hands around behind you to your feet, palms facing upward. Inhale as you do so.

● Focus on your breathing and encourage each breath to go deeply and fully into your back. Follow each inbreath with a long, soft outbreath.

▶　　　　　　▶　　**inhale**　　　　▶　　　　　‖

floor work
twist

The twist helps relieve tension and stiffness in the back, neck, and shoulders. As you perform the twist, you exercise the kidneys and abdominal organs, which helps improve digestion. This is a yoga breathing exercise.

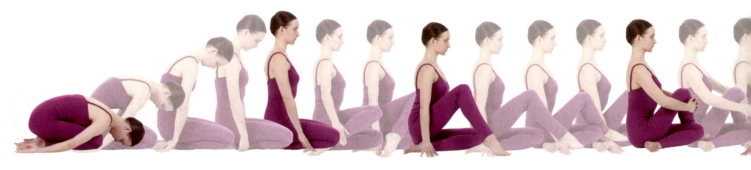

● Continue from the position on the previous page.

● Inhale as you unfold your body into an upright position.

● Drop over onto your left hip as you exhale. Bring your right leg over your left, pressing your right foot firmly into the floor on the outside of your left knee. The heel of your left foot should lay under your right hip. Press your sitting bones evenly into the floor.

● Inhale as you interlock your fingers and place your hands on your right shin, just below the knee.

▶ **inhale** ▶ **exhale** ▶ **inhale** ▶

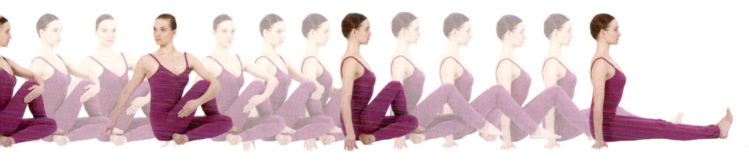

● Still inhaling, lift up through your hips and spine and lengthen the front of your body. Extend through the crown of your head toward the ceiling.

● Hook your left elbow around your right knee and place your left hand on the outside of the thigh. Place your right arm behind you, pressing your fingertips into the floor. Exhale as you lift and turn your trunk to the right. Hold for three to five breaths.

● Inhale as you release from the pose and come back to center, your hands on the floor either side of your hips.

● Stretch your legs out as you exhale, extending through your heels. Lift your spine and gaze ahead. Repeat on the other side.

▶ **exhale** ❙❙ ▶ **inhale** ▶ **exhale** ❙❙

sitting forward bend

This forward bend relieves fatigue and calms the mind. It also stretches and lengthens the spine and legs. If your hamstrings are tight, use a belt to loop around your feet (rather than using your hands) and do not fold forward. This is a yoga breathing exercise.

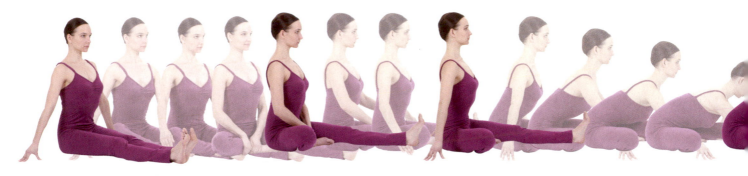

● Continue from the position on the previous page. Keep your hips anchored into the floor, your legs extending out in front of you and your trunk lifting. Inhale.

● Keeping your left leg straight, exhale as you bend your right knee out to the side. Use your hands to help you slide your right heel toward your groin. Press the sole of your foot against your left inner thigh.

● Inhale as you place your hands on either side of your hips, fingertips pressing into the ground. Lift and open your chest.

● As you exhale, hinge from your hips and extend your trunk forward and catch your left foot.

▶ **inhale**　　　　**exhale**　　　▶　　**inhale**　　　▶　　**exhale**　　　▶

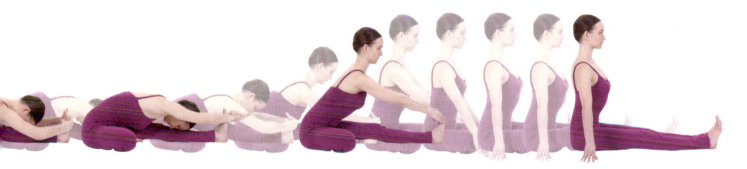

● Inhale as you extend your trunk.
Then exhale as you take your trunk
down over your left leg. Hold for
five breaths.

● If you have good flexibility, place
your hands around the ball of your
foot, your left hand around your right
wrist, and hold for five breaths. Keep
your upper back and shoulders wide,
your neck relaxed, and your elbows
lifting and extending to the sides.

● Inhale as you lift your head and
chest, extending through the front of
your body. Then exhale as you come
back up to sitting.

● Inhale as you stretch your right leg
out to join your left leg. Repeat on the
other side.

inhale and exhale ▶ ‖ ▶ **inhale and exhale** ▶ **inhale** ‖

wide leg stretch

The wide leg stretch brings flexibility to the hip sockets, inner thighs, and groin. It also boosts circulation to the pelvic area. Never force yourself to stretch further than is comfortable. If you wish to take the pressure off your knees, place rolled-up towels underneath them. Use yoga breathing.

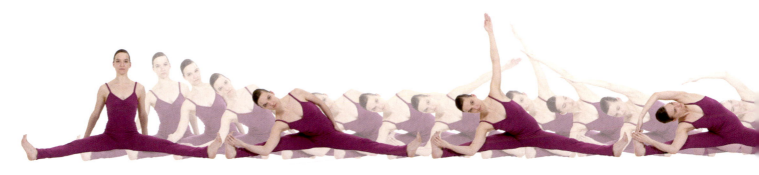

● Continue from the position on the previous page. Exhale as you take your legs out to the side as far as is comfortable. Inhale as you pull back the flesh on your buttocks so your weight is over your sitting bones.

● Keeping your hips anchored into the floor, exhale as you lower your right elbow onto the floor and hook the first two fingers of your right hand around your right big toe.

● Inhale as you press the backs of your legs down into the floor. Make sure you engage your pelvic floor and abdominals.

● Exhale as you lift your left arm up and over your head. If you can, catch the toes on your right foot. Turn your abdominals and chest toward the ceiling. Hold for five breaths.

▶ **exhale and inhale**   **exhale**   ▶   **inhale**   ▶   **exhale**   ❚❚ ▶

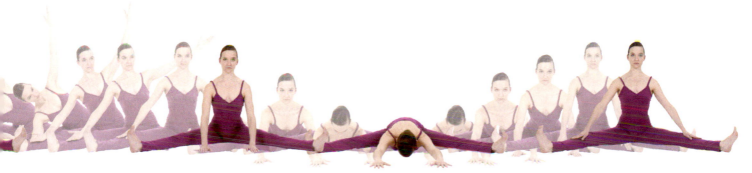

● Keep extending through both legs and root your hips down into the floor. Inhale as you smoothly come back to upright, your hands resting on your shins.

● As you exhale, place the palms of your hands on the floor in front of you. Keep both legs extending away evenly from your hips.

● Inhale as you lift and extend your trunk. Then exhale as you hinge from your hips and bring your body forward, leading with your chest. Only go as far as you can—never overstretch. Hold for five breaths, resting your body on the floor.

● Come back to upright as you inhale.

inhale   ▶   exhale   ▶   inhale and exhale   ❚❚ ▶   inhale   ❚❚

cobbler *work*

This stretch increases flexibility in the hips and knees. As well as stretching the spine, the weight of your head is used to release tension in the neck muscles. Place a cushion under your knees if you need extra support. This is a yoga breathing exercise.

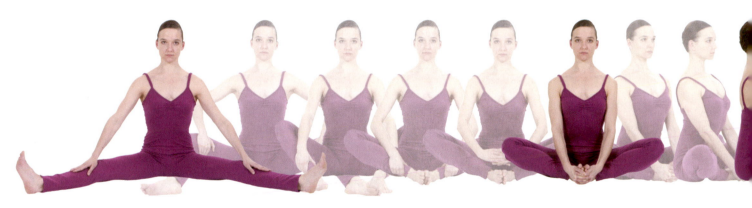

● Continue from the position on the previous page, sitting tall and looking straight ahead.

● Moving from a strong center, inhale as you place your hands under your knees. Lift them and start to draw the soles of your feet together.

● Exhale as you place your hands on your ankles and draw them toward your groin, the soles of your feet together.

● Interlock your fingers and place them under your feet.

▶   **inhale**   ▶   **exhale**   ▶   ▶

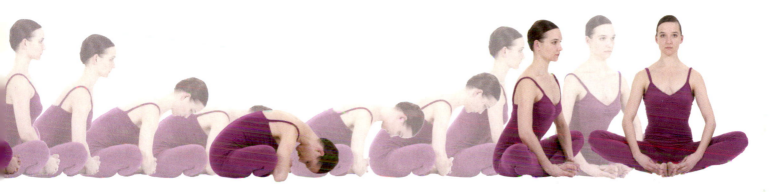

● Inhale as you lift and lengthen your trunk.

● With a strong abdominal contraction, exhale as you fold forward, your elbows in front of your shins. Only go as far as you can—do not overstretch. Keep your shoulders and upper back wide, your head heavy, and your neck relaxed. Hold for five breaths.

● Keeping your hips rooted into the floor, inhale as you extend your body back to upright.

● Exhale as you rest your hands on your feet.

inhale ▶ exhale ❚❚ ▶ inhale ▶ exhale ❚❚

floor work

hamstring stretch

The hamstring stretch brings flexibility to the hips and hamstrings. But avoid being tempted to overstretch—only go as far as is comfortable. The stretch can also be done by looping a belt around your foot, rather than using your hands. Breathe deeply into your hamstrings as you follow this sequence. Use yoga breathing.

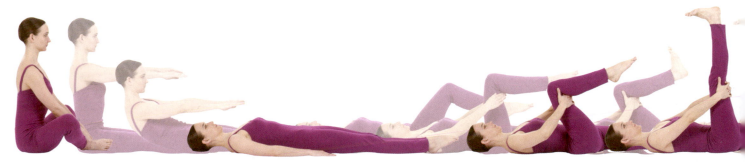

● Continue from the position on the previous page. Then from a firm base and strong center inhale as you stretch your legs out in front of you, extending through your ankles and toes. Also lift and extend your arms out in front of you.

● As you exhale, roll your spine down onto the floor, extending through your tailbone and drawing your abdominals in.

● Bring your right knee up, interlock your fingers, and place your hands on the back of your thigh. Inhale as you do so.

● As you exhale, flex your foot back and straighten your right leg toward the ceiling.

▶ **inhale**　　　　　**exhale**　　　▶　**inhale**　　　▶　**exhale**　　　▶

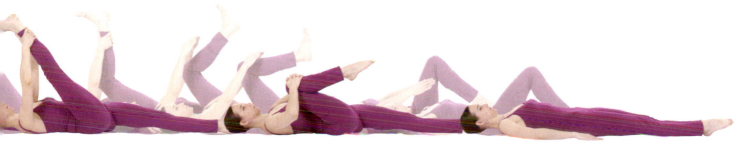

● Inhale as you slide your hands
down the back of your leg toward
your foot as far as is comfortable.
Exhale into your own full position.
Hold for five breaths.

● Release your leg, bend your knee,
and hug it to your chest as you inhale.
Keep your fingers interlocked. Hold for
two to three breaths.

● Exhale as you place your right foot
onto the floor.

● Straighten your right leg. Repeat on
the other side.

inhale and exhale   ‖ ▶   inhale   ‖ ▶   exhale   ▶   ‖

floor work

winding down

Winding down is a soothing and relaxing stretch for the back and waist. It is also designed to start

to calm the body into a state of relaxation. Use yoga breathing.

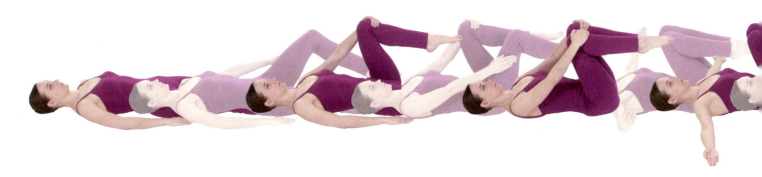

● Continue from the position on the previous page, both legs fully extended on the floor.

● Inhale as you slowly bring your left knee up to your chest, hooking your left hand around your shin.

● Follow this with the right knee, again hooking your right hand around your shin.

● With both hands on your shins, exhale and feel the weight of your head sinking into the floor.

►   **inhale**   ►   **exhale**   ►

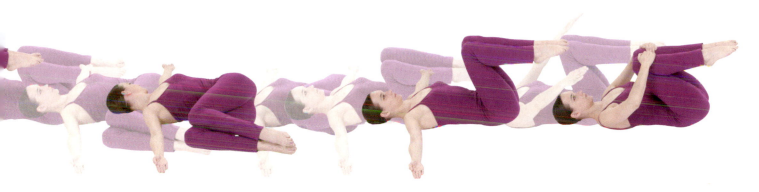

● Engage your pelvic floor and abdominals as you inhale. Move your arms out to the side at shoulder height, palms facing upward. Inhale as you do so.

● Exhale as you take your knees over toward your right elbow. Keep your upper back and shoulders wide, letting them drop into the floor. Slowly turn your head to the left. Release your pelvic floor and abdominals and let go of all tension. Hold for five breaths.

● Engage your pelvic floor and abdominals. Keeping your knees together, move from a strong center and inhale as you bring your legs back up to center.

● Exhale as you hug your knees; then inhale and hold. Exhale and repeat on the other side.

inhale ▶ exhale ❚❚ ▶ inhale ▶ exhale and inhale ❚❚

floor work

relaxation

Follow this sequence to relax after your yoga fusion practice and to allow the exercises you have just done to take full effect in the body. Keep a blanket handy to stay warm at the end. This is a yoga breathing exercise.

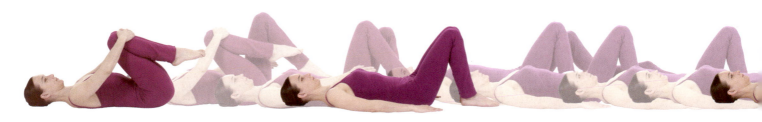

● Continue from the position on the previous page with your hands on your shins and your knees drawn into your chest.

● Exhale as you place your feet on the floor one at a time, hip width apart. Place your arms down by the sides of your body, palms facing downward.

● Slowly extend your right leg along the floor. Then slowly extend your left leg in the same way.

● Inhale as you extend your body, stretching through your fingers, toes, tailbone, and crown of your head. Turn your palms to face the ceiling. Relax and exhale.

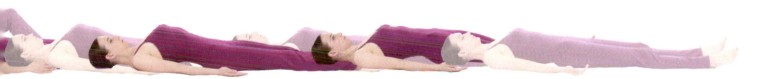

● Inhale as you lift your chest and slide your shoulder blades down your back. Relax and exhale.

● Inhale as you lift your hips slightly, extending your tailbone toward your feet. Exhale as you gently lower your hips back to the floor and completely relax your legs.

● Let all tension drain away and feel the weight of your body sink into the floor. Close your eyes and relax the muscles in your face. Release any tension in your neck.

● Close your mind down, acknowledging any thoughts or sounds, then letting them go. Surrender into deep relaxation. Breathe quietly and softly. Relax for five to ten minutes.

index